Development and Rational Use of Standardised MedDRA Queries (SMQs): Retrieving Adverse Drug Reactions with MedDRA

Report of the CIOMS SMQ Implementation Working Group

Second Edition

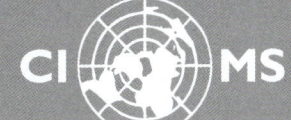

Copyright © 2016 by the Council for International Organizations of Medical Sciences (CIOMS)
ISBN 978-92-9036-086-5

All rights reserved. CIOMS publications may be obtained directly from:

CIOMS, P.O. Box 2100, CH-1211 Geneva 2, Switzerland, tel.: +41 22 791 6497, www.cioms.ch, e-mail: info@cioms.ch.

CIOMS publications are also available through the World Health Organization, WHO Press, 20 Avenue Appia, CH-1211 Geneva 27, Switzerland.

Citation for this document:

Development and rational use of standardised MedDRA queries (SMQs): Retrieving adverse drug reactions with MedDRA, Second Edition. Geneva: Council for International Organizations of Medical Sciences (CIOMS); 2016.

The authors alone are responsible for the views expressed in this publication and those views do not necessarily represent the decisions, policies or views of their respective institutions or companies.

Design and Layout: Paprika (Annecy, France)

ACKNOWLEDGEMENTS

The Council for International Organizations of Medical Sciences (CIOMS) gratefully acknowledges the contributions of the members of the CIOMS Implementation Working Group on Standardised MedDRA Queries (SMQs) for dedicating their time and providing their expertise to finalize this publication. Each member participated actively in the discussion, drafting and redrafting of texts and their review in order to bring the entire project to a successful conclusion.

Moreover, CIOMS recognizes the contribution of all members of the CIOMS SMQ Working Group and the CIOMS SMQ Core Group during the earlier stages, as well as the generous support of the regulatory authorities, pharmaceutical companies and other organizations and institutions which provided the expertise and resources that resulted in this publication.

CIOMS thanks especially those members who chaired the meetings for their capable leadership, and the rapporteurs for their dedication and professional contributions.

The editorial group, comprising Drs William Gregory, Ilona Grosse-Michaelis, Norbert Paeschke, Christina Winter and Ms Lynn Macdonald, merits special mention and thanks. CIOMS expresses special appreciation to Drs William Gregory and Ilona Grosse-Michaelis as Chief Editors of the final report.

The work has involved a number of meetings organized by the CIOMS Secretariat, and contributions from regulatory agencies and pharmaceutical companies that hosted the meetings (see Appendix 1) are especially acknowledged. At CIOMS Drs Gunilla Sjölin-Forsberg and Juhana E Idänpään-Heikkilä, Ms Amanda Owden, and Ms Sue le Roux managed the project. Ms Sue le Roux merits special thanks for contributing her editorial skills.

Gunilla Sjölin-Forsberg, MD, PhD
Former Secretary-General, CIOMS*

Juhana E Idänpään-Heikkilä[†], MD, PhD
Senior Adviser, CIOMS

Lembit Rägo, MD, PhD
Secretary-General, CIOMS

Geneva, Switzerland, April 2016

* Dr Gunilla Sjölin-Forsberg was Secretary-General of CIOMS from April 2010 to November 2015
† Dr Juhana E Idänpään-Heikkilä passed away on 10 October 2015.

DEDICATION

This report on Standardised MedDRA Queries (SMQs) is dedicated to the memory of the SMQ Working Groups' esteemed colleague, good friend and trusted adviser, Dr Juhana Idänpään-Heikkilä, who, as Secretary-General of CIOMS had the vision to organize a discussion of search strategies for adverse events in MedDRA-coded data, at Frankfurt airport in May 2002. This evolved into three successive SMQ Working Groups comprised of senior scientists from regulatory authorities, the biopharmaceutical industry, and other stakeholders. His experience, intelligence, and commitment were indispensable to the success of not only the SMQ Working Groups, but also the other CIOMS working groups that addressed many difficult issues related to pharmacovigilance and biomedical ethics.

Dr Heikkilä's important contributions to the field of pharmacovigilance are extensive and have left an indelible mark, not only through his work with CIOMS and the consensus process, but also from his participation in international scientific exchange and educational programmes. Dr Heikkilä served CIOMS for over 15 years; he was Secretary-General from 2000 to 2006 after which he served as Senior Adviser for nine years. Prior to his CIOMS tenure, Dr Heikkilä was Director of the Department of Drug Management and Policies at the World Health Organization in Geneva. During this entire time, Dr Heikkilä continued to fulfil his academic functions as Professor at the University of Helsinki Medical School faculty.

We hope that the usefulness of the second edition of "Development and Rational Use of Standardised MedDRA Queries (SMQs): Retrieving Adverse Drug Reactions with MedDRA" in practical settings will benefit the safety of patients and will meet the high ethical and professional standards Dr Heikkilä set for himself.

Dr Heikkilä passed away on 10 October 2015; he will be sorely missed by all who knew him.

TABLE OF CONTENTS

ACKNOWLEDGEMENTS iii

DEDICATION iv

INITIALISMS AND GLOSSARY.. xi

PREFACE xvii

DISCLAIMERS AND CLARIFICATIONS xix

CHAPTER I. INTRODUCTION 1
Executive summary 1
I.A. Origins of SMQs 1
I.B. Overview of purpose and content of this publication 3
I.C. Target audience 3

CHAPTER II. OVERVIEW OF SMQ CONCEPTS 5
Executive summary 5
II.A. SMQ definition 5
II.B. SMQ benefits and limitations...5
II.C. SMQ applications...6
II.D. Development of SMQs 7
II.E. MedDRA Version Analysis Tool (MVAT)...7
II.F. SMQ design features 8
II.G. SMQ modifications and organization-specific queries 10
II.H. SMQ maintenance 11
II.I. Consideration of requests for new SMQs 11
II.J. Testing of SMQs..12
II.K. Summary of concepts and proposals for use of SMQs......................14

CHAPTER III. SEARCH STRATEGIES WITH A FOCUS ON PHARMACOVIGILANCE ..15

Executive summary 15
III.A. Introduction 15
III.B. General considerations for search strategies 17
III.C. Communication and documentation of the search strategy...................................19
III.D. Limitations – guidelines to avoid pitfalls..22
III.E. Customized searches 25
III.F. Conclusions and recommendations 25

CHAPTER IV. TECHNICAL ASPECTS OF IMPLEMENTATION 27

Executive summary 27
IV.A. Introduction 27
IV.B. Practical guidance for implementing SMQs 27
IV.C. How to deal with algorithms 33
IV.D. Algorithmic SMQs using weight factors 35
IV.E. Conclusions and recommendations 38

CHAPTER V. COMMUNICATION OF RESULTS 39

Executive summary 39
V.A. General considerations for communication of search results 39
V.B. Points to consider when preparing a report with query output 39
V.C. Conclusions and recommendations 42

CHAPTER VI. CURRENT CONSIDERATIONS AND FUTURE DIRECTIONS 43

Executive summary 43
VI.A. Current considerations 43
VI.B. Future directions...44

APPENDICES 47

APPENDIX 1. MEMBERSHIP AND WORKING PROCEDURES OF THE CIOMS SMQ WORKING GROUPS 49

APPENDIX 2. EXAMPLES OF SMQ DEVELOPMENT 57
APPENDIX 2.a. Example of SMQ development: SMQ *Rhabdomyolysis/myopathy* 58
- A.2.a.A. Background on rhabdomyolysis and myopathy 58
- A.2.a.B. Methodology 58
- A.2.a.C. Results 59
- A.2.a.D. Summary and conclusions...60

APPENDIX 2.b. Example of SMQ development: SMQ *Anaphylactic reaction* 67
- A.2.b.A. Definition and background 67
- A.2.b.B. Methodology 67
- A.2.b.C. Algorithmic approach...68
- A.2.b.D. Results of testing 68
- A.2.b.E. Summary and conclusions...69

APPENDIX 2.c. Example of SMQ development: SMQ *Hepatic disorders*......................77
- A.2.c.A. Introduction.. 77
- A.2.c.B. Overview of SMQ *Hepatic disorders* 77
- A.2.c.C. Search strategy.. 79
- A.2.c.D. Specifications 81
- A.2.c.E. Pre-release testing 88
- A.2.c.F. Modifications of SMQ *Hepatic disorders* over time 96
- A.2.c.G. Tabulation of PTs listed for SMQ *Hepatic disorders* MedDRA v8.0 and v18.0..99

APPENDIX 3. COMMUNICATION OF SEARCH RESULTS 115

LIST OF TABLES

Table II.F.1. Two examples of algorithmic SMQs 10

Table III.D.1. Broad terms excluded because they are in the SMQs *Peripheral neuropathy* and/or *Guillain-Barre syndrome* (MedDRA v10.1) 23

Table III.D.2. Broad terms excluded because they are nonspecific, related to advanced demyelination, or did not test well during SMQ development (MedDRA v10.1) 24

Table IV.B.1. Example for output of SOC hierarchy for a given PT 28

Table IV.B.2. Example for output of a case safety report 28

Table IV.B.3. Example for output of SOC hierarchy for a given PT linked to a case report 28

Table IV.B.4. Representation of hierarchical levels in the SMQ list file 29

Table IV.B.5. Example for data output from the SMQ content file 30

Table IV.B.6. Structure and source fields of a combined file of SMQ list and content file resulting in an SMQ hierarchy file 31

Table IV.B.7. SMQ hierarchical information linked to case data 32

Table IV.C.1. Information about term category and scope linked to case data 33

Table IV.C.2. Example for a subset of data 33

Table IV.C.3. Spreadsheet of example data, count of terms by category per case report 34

Table IV.D.1. Example for subset of data for SMQ *Systemic lupus erythematosus* 35

Table IV.D.2. Spreadsheet of example data, sum of weight factors by category per case report..37

Table A.1.1. Milestones for SMQ development by the CIOMS Working Group, as of November 2004 (with subsequent modification) 50

Table A.1.2. Members, advisors and observers who have contributed to the development of SMQs as part of the CIOMS SMQ Working Groups (2002–2016) 50

Table A.1.3. Face-to-face meetings of the CIOMS SMQ Working Group, CIOMS SMQ Core Group, and CIOMS SMQ Implementation Working Group, as of September 2015 54

Table A.2.a.1. SMQ *Rhabdomyolysis/myopathy*-related PTs for narrow search 61

Table A.2.a.2. SMQ *Rhabdomyolysis/myopathy*-related PTs for broad search 61

Table A.2.a.3. Health-care professional, nonclinical study cases reporting SMQ *Rhabdomyolysis/myopathy*-related MedDRA PTs for two test products reported to testing company's safety database during the time periods under review 63

Table A.2.a.4. Number of nonclinical study cases reported by health-care professionals identified by narrow and broad search for SMQ *Rhabdomyolysis/myopathy*-related events 65

Table A.2.a.5. Number of nonclinical study cases reported by health-care professionals identified by search for SMQ *Rhabdomyolysis/myopathy*-related events, further categorized by the presence of other PTs reported in the same case 65

Table A.2.b.1. Post-marketing cases reporting anaphylactic reaction-related MedDRA PTs for three test products reported to the regulator from 1 January 1998 to 1 January 2004 (MedDRA v7.0) 70

Table A.2.b.2. Summary of narrow search, broad search and algorithmic approach of post-marketing cases reporting anaphylactic reaction-related MedDRA PTs for three test products reported to the regulator from 1 January 1998 to 1 January 2004 (MedDRA v7.0) 72

Table A.2.b.3. Cases reporting anaphylactic reaction-related MedDRA PTs for three pharmaceutical company test products from 1 January 1980 to 1 January 2004 (MedDRA v7.0) 73

Table A.2.b.4. Summary of narrow search, broad search and algorithmic approach of cases reporting anaphylactic reaction-related MedDRA PTs for three test products reported to the pharmaceutical company from 1 January 1980 to 1 January 2004 (MedDRA v7.0) 75

Table A.2.c.1. Summary topics of SMQ *Hepatic disorders* 79

Table A.2.c.2. Adverse event and co-manifestation PTs belonging to the searches for possible drug-induced liver toxicity of four test products entered onto company A's drug safety database up to 19 February 2004, MedDRA v6.1 91

Table A.2.c.3. Cases identified by searches 3.1 and 3.2 95

Table A.2.c.4. Odds ratios calculated for percentage of events of possible drug-related liver toxicity searches for five test compounds compared to the entire database, MedDRA v6.1 96

Table A.2.c.5. Renaming within SMQ *Hepatic disorders* 97

Table A.2.c.6. Examples of PT changes in SMQ *Hepatic disorders* from initial publication to MedDRA v18.0 98

Table A.2.c.7. Tabulation of PTs listed for SMQ *Hepatic disorders*, MedDRA v8.0 and v18.0 100

Table A.3.1. Communication of search results 115

LIST OF FIGURES

Figure I.A.1. MedDRA hierarchy of terms 2

Figure II.F.1. Depiction of two types of SMQ 9

Figure II.F.2. Depiction of a hierarchical SMQ 9

Figure III.A.1. Hierarchical structure of SMQ *Cardiac arrhythmias* (MedDRA v18.0) 16

Figure IV.B.1. Hierarchical structure of SMQ *Hepatic disorders* (MedDRA v18.0) 29

Figure IV.B.2. Relation between SMQ list and content file to extract hierarchy information 30

Figure A.2.c.1. Graphical overview of SMQ *Hepatic disorders* (MedDRA v18.0) 78

INITIALISMS AND GLOSSARY

This list of initialisms and the glossary contain key terms used in this report. Most of these terms have been in common use for some time but, in spite of various international consensus initiatives, certain terms in the glossary do not have universally-accepted definitions. The glossary is not intended to be comprehensive but rather is intended to provide relevant terms and associated definitions as used in this report.

Note that each published SMQ has an associated CIOMS- and ICH-endorsed definition in the explanatory material published by the MSSO.

INITIALISMS

BfArM	Federal Institute for Drugs and Medical Devices (Germany)
CG	Core Group
CIOMS	Council for International Organizations of Medical Sciences
CK	Creatine kinase
CK-MM	Isoform originating skeletal muscle
CRO	Contract research organization
DME	Designated medical event
DSUR	Development Safety Update Report
EMEA	European Medicines Agency
HLGT	High Level Group Term
HLT	High Level Term
ICD	International Classification of Diseases
ICH	International Council for Harmonisation of Technical Requirements for Pharmaceuticals for Human Use (formerly International Conference on Harmonisation of Technical Requirements for Registration of Pharmaceuticals for Human Use)
ICSR	Individual Case Safety Report
IFPMA	International Federation of Pharmaceutical Manufacturers and Associations
IWG	Implementation Working Group
JMO	Japanese Maintenance Organization
LLT	Lowest Level Term
MAG	MedDRA Analytical Grouping
MedDRA	Medical Dictionary for Regulatory Activities
MHRA	Medicines and Healthcare products Regulatory Agency (UK)
MMB	MedDRA Management Board
MPA	Medical Products Agency (Sweden)

MSSO	MedDRA Maintenance and Support Services Organization
MVAT	MedDRA Version Analysis Tool
NEC	Not elsewhere classified
NOS	Not otherwise specified
PBRER	Periodic Benefit–Risk Evaluation Report
PSUR	Periodic Safety Update Report
PT	Preferred Term
SLE	Systemic lupus erythematosus
SMQ	Standardised MedDRA Query
SOC	System Organ Class
SQL	Structured query language
SSC	Special Search Category
SSQ	Standardised Search Query
v	version
vs.	versus
WG	Working Group
WHO	World Health Organization
WHO-ART	WHO-Adverse Reaction Terminology

GLOSSARY

Active SMQ

An active SMQ (or sub-SMQ) is included with the current version of MedDRA. The terms in an active SMQ are maintained in step with each version of MedDRA and are categorized either as "active" or "inactive".

Ad hoc MedDRA query

A MedDRA query designed to support a search not defined by a published SMQ. An ad hoc query may be created de novo in instances when an existing SMQ does not cover the medical condition of interest. Ad hoc queries are maintained outside the ICH/CIOMS process and are not considered SMQs. The concept of an ad hoc query is similar to a "modified SMQ" or "customized SMQ" (i.e. an ad hoc query is not an SMQ).

Adverse event (AE) (USA synonym: Adverse experience)

Any untoward medical occurrence in a patient or clinical investigation subject administered a pharmaceutical product which does not necessarily have a causal relationship with this treatment. Note: An adverse event can therefore be any unfavourable and unintended sign (including an abnormal laboratory finding), symptom or disease temporally associated with the use of a medicinal (investigational) product, whether or not related to the medicinal (investigational) product. [1, 2]

References:
1. ICH E6(R1) guideline. Guideline for good clinical practice, E6(R1). Step 4, 10 June 2006 (including post-step 4 corrections). Geneva: International Conference on Harmonisation; 2006.
2. Practical aspects of signal detection in pharmacovigilance. Report of the CIOMS Working Group VIII. Geneva: CIOMS; 2010.

Adverse (drug) reaction

A noxious and unintended response to a medicinal product for which there is a reasonable possibility that the product caused the response. The phrase "response to a medicinal product" means that a causal relationship between a medicinal product and an adverse event is at least a reasonable possibility. The phrase "a reasonable possibility" means that there are facts, evidence, or arguments to support a causal association with the medicinal product. Note: From a regulatory perspective, all spontaneous reports are considered "suspected" adverse drug reactions in that they convey the suspicions of the reporters. A causality assessment by the regulatory authority may indicate whether there could be alternative explanations for the observed adverse event other than the suspect drug. It should be noted that although overdose is not included in the basic definition of an adverse (drug) reaction in the post-approval environment, information regarding overdose, abuse and misuse should be included as part of the risk assessment of any medicinal product. [3, 4]

References:
3. ICH E2A guideline. Clinical safety data management: definitions and standards for expedited reporting. Step 4. Geneva: International Conference on Harmonisation; 2006.
4. Practical aspects of signal detection in pharmacovigilance. Report of the CIOMS Working Group VIII. Geneva: CIOMS; 2010.

Algorithmic SMQ

This is a design feature that employs a stepwise (algorithmic) approach to a standardised query. Note: For these SMQs, broad-scope terms are further subdivided into categories of similar terms and designated as Category B, Category C, etc. Narrow terms are always Category A for algorithmic SMQs. The theory behind an algorithmic SMQ is that a case is more likely to be of interest if it contains a defined combination of broad terms than if it contains any one broad term. The intention behind algorithmic designs is to reduce "noise" when applied to a large database.

Broad search strategy/Broad SMQ/Broad scope

A broad SMQ contains terms that are less specific for the condition of interest and may retrieve events of interest, but may also retrieve some data that are not relevant and only introduce "noise" in the search results.

Customized SMQ

A customized SMQ is the query resulting from modification of a published SMQ (or sub-SMQ) to address user needs that are not met by the published query. MedDRA terms may be added or deleted from the published query. The concept of a customized SMQ is similar to a "modified SMQ" or an ad hoc query (i.e. it is not an SMQ). See Ad hoc MedDRA query and Modified SMQ.

Designated medical event (DME)

Adverse events considered rare, serious, and associated with a high drug-attributable risk and which constitute an alarm with as few as one to three reports. Examples include Stevens-Johnson syndrome, toxic epidermal necrolysis, hepatic failure, anaphylaxis, aplastic anaemic and torsade de pointes. [5]

References:
5. Hauben M et al. The role of data mining in pharmacovigilance. Expert Opin Drug Saf. 2005; 4:929–48.

Event of Interest

The medical condition defined in SMQ documentation (or in documentation for an ad hoc query, a customized SMQ, or a modified SMQ).

ICH MedDRA Advisory Panel

A committee that represents the ICH Parties and provides a liaison between the CIOMS SMQ Working Groups (WGs) and the ICH MedDRA Management Board. The panel must endorse new work items before the CIOMS WG begins work and must also endorse candidate SMQs and documentation for the ICH MMB before production by the MSSO/JMO.

Individual case safety report (ICSR)

A report of information describing adverse event(s)/reaction(s) experienced by an individual patient. The event(s)/reaction(s) can be related to the administration of one or more medicinal products at a particular point in time. The ICSR can also be used for exchange of other information, such as medication error(s) that do not involve adverse event(s)/reaction(s). [6] ICSR is often used as a synonym for adverse (drug) reaction report.

References:
6. ICH E2B (R3) implementation guide, clinical safety data management: data elements for transmission of individual case safety reports. Geneva: International Conference on Harmonisation; version 5.01, April 2015. (Also see ISO/HL7 27953-2:2011 International standard, Health informatics – Individual case safety reports (ICSRs) in pharmacovigilance – part 2: Human pharmaceutical reporting requirements for ICSR).

Inactive SMQ

An inactive SMQ is one that will no longer be maintained with successive versions of MedDRA. The terms in an inactive SMQ are "frozen" as of the most recent version of the previously active SMQ. An SMQ (or sub-SMQ) may be made inactive if it has been found not to be useful to users, becomes outdated, or is found to be otherwise problematic. If the original rationale for the query remains valid, the inactive SMQ may be replaced by a newly developed, more comprehensive, or more clearly structured query with a modified name. See Inactive SMQ term.

Inactive SMQ term

MedDRA PTs in an SMQ that have been made inactive in that SMQ. The SMQ may be either active or inactive. These terms are retained in their SMQ and are not deleted. An "inactive" status may be assigned if the term is found to have been included in error, if the inclusion criteria of the SMQ changed, or if justified by changes in medical or regulatory science or due to restructuring of the SMQ. If an LLT is moved to a PT that is not part of the SMQ, it will also be made inactive. This concept of "inactive" is different from the concept of "non-current" as applied only to coding with LLTs. When applying an SMQ for data retrieval, inactive LLTs and PTs should be removed from the search.

Level-1 SMQ

The most comprehensive query for the condition of interest (i.e. a level-1 SMQ) includes all sub-SMQs (e.g. SMQ levels 2, 3, 4 and 5, as relevant) under the named SMQ.

Level-2 (or 3 or 4 or 5) SMQ

Sub-SMQs that are subsumed under a level-1 SMQ.

Modified SMQ

A modified SMQ is the query resulting from addition or deletion of MedDRA terms from a published SMQ (or sub-SMQ) which is modified to address user needs that are not met by the published query. The concept of a modified SMQ is the same as a "customized SMQ" or an ad hoc query (i.e. it is not an SMQ). See Ad hoc MedDRA query and Customized SMQ.

Narrow search strategy/Narrow SMQ/Narrow scope

A query with MedDRA terms that are constrained to those highly likely to represent the condition of interest and, therefore, confer specificity to the results of the search. A narrow search includes only the narrow terms, in contrast to a broad search which includes all the terms in the SMQ, i.e. narrow scope terms plus broad scope terms.

Pharmacovigilance

The science and activities relating to the detection, assessment, understanding and prevention of adverse effects or any other drug-related problem. [7]

References:
7. The importance of pharmacovigilance – safety monitoring of medicinal products. Geneva: World Health Organization; 2002:42 (Glossary).

READ

READ codes are the standard clinical terminology system used in General Practice in the United Kingdom. They provide detailed clinical encoding of multiple patient phenomena including diagnoses and clinical signs and symptoms, further clinical observations, laboratory tests and results, performed procedures (diagnostic, therapeutic or surgical), as well as a variety of administrative items (e.g. whether a screening recall has been sent, by what communication modality, or whether an item of service fee has been claimed) and further information about social circumstances, occupation, ethnicity and religion. They therefore include but go significantly beyond the expressivity of a diagnosis coding system.

Signal

Information that arises from one or multiple sources (including observations and experiments), which suggests a new potentially causal association or a new aspect of a known association, between an intervention and an event or set of related events, either adverse or beneficial, that is judged to be of sufficient likelihood to justify verification. [8]

References:
8. Practical aspects of signal detection in pharmacovigilance. Report of CIOMS Working Group VIII. Geneva: CIOMS; 2010.

Standardised MedDRA Query (SMQ)

SMQs are groups of MedDRA PTs that focus on a defined medical condition. They are designed as a supplement to the MedDRA hierarchy for identifying and retrieving MedDRA-coded data, e.g. ICSRs, that are potentially relevant to the condition of interest. SMQs are maintained with each version of MedDRA. Note: Each SMQ may have active and inactive PTs for a given SMQ. The designation of a PT as inactive for an SMQ does not necessarily correlate with the designation of a MedDRA LLT as "non-current".

Sub-SMQ

In hierarchical SMQs, a sub-SMQ is a stand-alone standard query categorized at levels 2, 3, 4 or 5.

PREFACE

The CIOMS Working Groups (WGs) within the area of drug safety have evolved over the years. A broad range of challenging drug safety topics have been addressed by these Working Groups, which comprised expert senior scientists from regulatory authorities, the biopharmaceutical industry and academia. These experts have developed consensus guidelines and pragmatic recommendations in important public health areas.

From the beginning the WGs focused on the processes for detection and management of potential problems during the development and use of drugs. The initial guidelines for international reporting of safety information/adverse events with a standardised CIOMS I form were followed by guidance on Periodic Safety Update Reports (PSURs) and core data sheets.

Initially the WGs concentrated on post-authorization processes but as new WGs were formed, the scope was widened to include safety aspects of the whole life cycle of medicinal products. [1, 2, 3, 4] The reports of CIOMS WG V, [5] WG VI [6] and WG VII [7] covered areas such as pragmatic approaches in pharmacovigilance, management of safety information from clinical trials, and harmonisation of the format and content for PSURs during clinical trials – i.e. the Development Safety Update Report (DSUR). This was followed by the CIOMS WG VIII report [8] on signal detection, managing the life cycle of a signal including detection, prioritization and evaluation of a signal. The next report in the series, the CIOMS WG IX report, presents practical approaches to risk minimization. [9] A subsequent report prepared by the CIOMS WG X presents considerations for systematic reviews of clinical safety data. [10]

As the CIOMS WGs have no legal jurisdiction or mandate to make binding decisions, reliance is placed on other bodies to incorporate the CIOMS recommendations, guidelines or good practices into a regulatory or legislative framework. In many instances the reports of the CIOMS Working Groups have served as the basis for International Council for Harmonisation[A] (ICH) topics, and have either been included as such or with changes, or are referenced in ICH topics that have been included into legal frameworks governing the development and use of medicinal products in the European Union, Japan, USA and elsewhere.

The WGs on SMQs are unique in more than one aspect. Apart from the 2004 published report *SMQs development and rational use of standardised MedDRA queries (SMQs): Retrieving adverse drug reactions with MedDRA,* [11] there has been continuous development of SMQs by the members ongoing for over 12 years. This CIOMS activity has been conducted in conjunction with the ICH MedDRA Management Board (MMB). The CIOMS WG was initially established following an organizational meeting in May 2002 and the original 24 members were senior scientists representing seven regulatory authorities, seven pharmaceutical companies, and other organizations (e.g. World Health Organization [WHO] and CIOMS). Subsequently, a joint initiative of the MedDRA Maintenance and Support Services Organization (MSSO) and the Japanese Maintenance Organization (JMO), which had similar ambitions for the MedDRA terminology, was launched to take full advantage of technical expertise. In order to have a uniform approach to SMQ development, documentation and testing, the WG developed and implemented a consistent facilitation process that included testing in regulatory and company safety databases. Following several years of work the WG's activities were streamlined and the group first became a Core Group and later on an Implementation Working Group (IWG).

SMQs represent a standardised approach to establishing a baseline for the identification of Individual Case Safety Reports (ICSRs) that may represent defined medical conditions with the potential to have an impact on benefit–risk evaluations. Examples of the valuable use of SMQs, such as monitoring of potential safety risks and analysis of aggregate data, are included in this report. These examples are meant to illustrate the use of queries in systematic analyses (e.g. meta-analysis), interventional clinical trials, signal detection, signal assessment, and other database searches. In clinical trials, SMQs can be used to compare test medical product to comparators, including placebo, and to other molecules in the same class or with a

---

[A] In full: International Council for Harmonisation of Technical Requirements for Pharmaceuticals for Human Use, formerly known as the International Conference on Harmonisation. In October 2015, the International Conference on Harmonisation (ICH) underwent an organizational change, which saw it renamed the International Council for Harmonisation (ICH).

similar mechanism of action. SMQs can also serve as useful tools in vaccine vigilance and technovigilance (medical devices).

In Chapter I there is an introduction to the purpose and content of this report as well as a description of the origin of SMQs. In Chapter II the benefits and applications of SMQs are addressed in addition to their limitations. Structural design features are described, including narrow, broad, hierarchical and algorithmic scope. Chapter III deals with search strategies focusing on pharmacovigilance. General considerations on communication of search results are discussed in Chapter V, while Chapter VI presents the compiled recommendations of the IWG as well as future directions. At the end of the report some useful examples of SMQ development have been included in the appendices. In the future, there may also be opportunities to apply SMQs to active safety surveillance and non-interventional studies, as for instance the use of SMQ concepts in grouping International Classification of Diseases (ICD) and other codes.

References:

1. International reporting of adverse drug reactions. Report of CIOMS Working Group I (including Suspect Adverse Reaction Report Form – CIOMS Form I). Geneva: CIOMS; 1990.
2. International reporting of periodic drug safety update summaries. Report of CIOMS Working Group II. Geneva: CIOMS; 1993.
3. Guidelines for preparing core clinical safety information on drugs. Report of CIOMS Working Group III. Geneva: CIOMS; 1995.
4. Benefit–risk balance for marketed drugs: evaluating safety signals. Report of CIOMS Working Group IV. Geneva: CIOMS; 1998.
5. Guidelines for preparing core clinical safety information on drugs, second edition. Report of CIOMS Working Groups III and V. Geneva: CIOMS; 1999.
6. Management of safety information from clinical trials. Report of CIOMS Working Group VI. Geneva: CIOMS; 2005.
7. Development Safety Update Report (DSUR): harmonizing the format and content for periodic safety reporting during clinical trials. Report of CIOMS Working Group VII. Geneva: CIOMS; 2006.
8. Practical aspects of signal detection in pharmacovigilance. Report of CIOMS Working Group VIII. Geneva: CIOMS; 2010.
9. Practical approaches to risk minimisation for medicinal products. Report of CIOMS Working Group IX. Geneva: CIOMS; 2014.
10. Considerations for applying good meta-analysis practices to clinical safety data within the biopharmaceutical regulatory process. Report of CIOMS Working Group X. Geneva: CIOMS; 2016.
11. Development and rational use of standardised MedDRA queries (SMQs): retrieving adverse drug reactions with MedDRA. Report of the CIOMS SMQ Working Group, first edition. Geneva: CIOMS; 2004.

DISCLAIMERS AND CLARIFICATIONS

This publication includes three candidate SMQs developed by the WG, namely SMQ *Rhabdomyolysis/ myopathy*, SMQ *Anaphylactic reaction* and SMQ *Hepatic disorders*. It should be stressed that they are published only as examples to illustrate the structure and content of the end-product (i.e. SMQs) and are by no means intended to be incorporated into any system or used routinely as search queries.

MedDRA is used consistently without the trademark ® throughout this report.

MedDRA users should be aware that the MedDRA terminology changes twice yearly (MedDRA versions x.0 and x.1); therefore always check the MedDRA version number particularly for the examples. The respective MedDRA version information is updated as appropriate for each new MedDRA version. The documents are on the MedDRA homepage www.meddra.org but mainly those relating to the latest and more recent MedDRA versions. If MedDRA users require the documentation for the previous versions, they should send a specific request to MSSO. Always check the current MedDRA/SMQ version as there are changes over time.

Italics have been used throughout the document for SMQ and MedDRA hierarchical content with the exception that no italics are used within tables.

MedDRA subscribers and users are used synonymously throughout the document related to their actions according to the SMQ usage. Medical or medicinal is another example of synonymously used wording.

Throughout this report, unless indicated otherwise, the term "drug" is meant to include all medicines (e.g. drugs, vaccines, biotechnology products) for prevention, prophylaxis or treatment of a disease or medical condition, and possibly for use in diagnosis.

Important topics are repeated in different chapters, allowing readers to focus on specific chapters only.

Members of the CIOMS SMQ WGs have contributed their views and technical expertise and these do not necessarily represent the views of their respective organizations.

CHAPTER I.

INTRODUCTION

Executive summary

The MedDRA[A] subscriber community, including health authorities, recognized the need for a standard approach to identify and retrieve adverse events of interest from MedDRA-coded databases. Beginning in 2002, several strategies to address this need developed independently but the strategies eventually converged and a collaborative effort was eventually undertaken by CIOMS, the International Conference for Harmonisation of Technical Requirements for Pharmaceuticals for Human Use (ICH), and the MedDRA Maintenance and Support Services Organization (MSSO) to develop, publish, and maintain Standardised MedDRA Queries (SMQ).

I.A. Origins of SMQs

During its many years of existence, one of the roles of CIOMS has been to take up contentious research ethics issues as well as issues related to drug safety and drug development.

CIOMS has provided a neutral forum to facilitate development of consensus on how to resolve these issues through specially organized Working Groups comprising senior scientists who are members of interested parties and stakeholders. This role of serving as a neutral platform for the public and private sectors as well as for the scientific community has proved its utility on many occasions in the past.

A similar approach was also initially considered for the development of SMQs. Historically, the project with the practical suggestions described in this publication began as a CIOMS initiative. This was in response to suggestions from several regulatory authorities and pharmaceutical companies that there was a need to develop standard term lists for specific disease-based search programs based on MedDRA.

MedDRA was developed by the ICH and is used widely by regulatory authorities, the pharmaceutical and biotechnology industries, and academia for coding, reporting, analysing and communicating regulatory and safety information in pharmacovigilance databases for drugs (or biopharmaceuticals) and other medical and health products (e.g. vaccines). MedDRA is organized into a five-tiered hierarchy of terms that represent medical conditions, indications, investigations, medical and surgical procedures, medication errors, product quality terms, pharmacogenetic terms, toxicological terms, product defect terms, medical device-related issues, and terms to record medical and social histories. As of MedDRA v19.0, the terms are organized into 27 System Organ Classes (SOCs) that are further subdivided into groupings – High Level Group Terms (HLGTs) and High Level Terms (HLTs). HLTs group together unique medical concepts called Preferred Terms (PTs) to which are linked Lowest Level Terms (LLTs), which are generally synonyms of their parent PTs. Each PT term also appears as an LLT term in the hierarchy. Natural language information, i.e. the reporter's "verbatim", is often linked to individual LLTs and stored in user databases. This is illustrated in Figure 1.A.1, with examples and information on the number of categories at each level in the category.

[A] Medical Dictionary for Regulatory Activities is a product of ICH.

Figure I.A.1. MedDRA hierarchy of terms

MedDRA Hierarchy of Terms *
Abbreviation ( ) & Number [ ] in MedDRA v16.0
& Example at each level

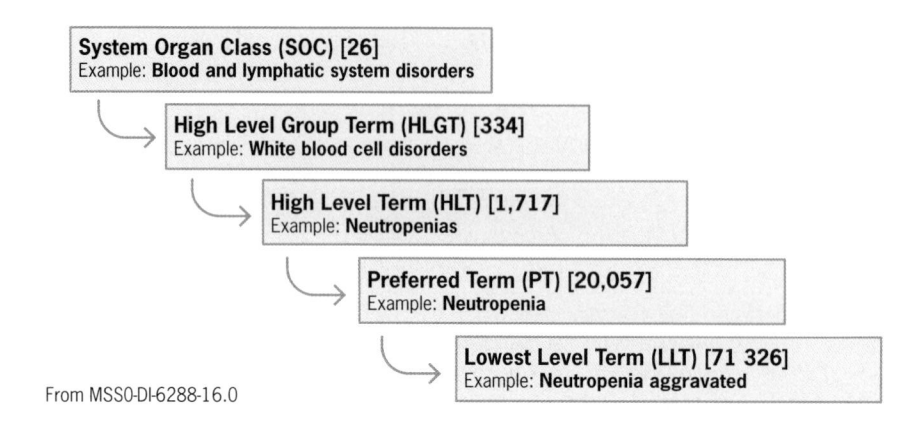

System Organ Class (SOC) [26]
Example: **Blood and lymphatic system disorders**

↳ **High Level Group Term (HLGT) [334]**
Example: **White blood cell disorders**

↳ **High Level Term (HLT) [1,717]**
Example: **Neutropenias**

↳ **Preferred Term (PT) [20,057]**
Example: **Neutropenia**

↳ **Lowest Level Term (LLT) [71 326]**
Example: **Neutropenia aggravated**

From MSSO-DI-6288-16.0

---

* This figure is valid for the MedDRA version given, but please see also the current MedDRA/SMQ version.

New versions of the MedDRA terminology are released each March and September in eleven languages. For more information on the scope and structure of MedDRA, refer to the *MedDRA introductory guide*. [1]

Without a standardised framework for a query, the size, granularity and complexity of MedDRA could result in different users selecting differing sets of terms related to a specific suspected drug-associated event. This may lead to retrieval of different ICSRs that are relevant to the event of interest.

SMQs arose out of a recognized need of the MedDRA subscriber community for a standard approach to assist in the identification and retrieval of MedDRA-coded safety data that may be helpful in addressing a specific safety question. The original MedDRA Special Search Categories (SSCs) were intended for a similar purpose, but after several years of MedDRA use the biopharmaceutical community (regulators and industry) concluded that these tools did not adequately address the need. In response, the MSSO began to develop MedDRA Analytical Groupings (MAGs) which were collections of terms from the MedDRA hierarchy that were related to medical conditions of interest.

At the same time, an independent initiative by CIOMS was started to address the need for special queries and groupings of terms to identify medical concepts of interest using MedDRA-coded data; their groupings were called Standardised Search Queries (SSQs). It was clear that the concepts of MAGs and SSQs were quite similar to one another and were both intended to fulfil the perceived need for retrieval tools to accompany MedDRA. Thus, CIOMS and ICH agreed that it was in the user community's best interest for the CIOMS Working Group and the MSSO to combine their efforts in developing these tools under the governance of the MedDRA Management Board (MMB). To recognize the joint effort, the former "MAG" and "SSQ" designations were discontinued, and an agreement on a name for these new standard groupings was reached. Since May 2003, work products resulting from the joint efforts of the CIOMS WG and MSSO have been designated SMQs. In November 2003, the ICH MMB endorsed the cooperative effort for the development of SMQs with an ICH MedDRA Advisory Panel providing liaison between the CIOMS WG and ICH.

The CIOMS SMQ WGs have been composed of senior scientists from several regulatory authorities, international pharmaceutical companies, the MSSO, the Japanese Maintenance Organization (JMO), WHO, and other institutions. Experts were selected for the WG from stakeholder organizations to represent a fair balance and so that no constituency would have a preponderance of influence. The WG also collaborates with other groups involved in similar activities, such as the CIOMS WG on the Pharmacovigilance of Vaccines and the Brighton Collaboration.

At the time of the introduction of MedDRA v18.0, there were 98 SMQ topics (level-1 SMQs) available that contain within them 116 sub-SMQs (hierarchical SMQs).

I.B. Overview of purpose and content of this publication

The aim of this CIOMS publication is to inform regulatory authorities, scientific institutions, pharmaceutical companies, and other organizations or individuals involved in biopharmaceutical and other medical product development about the purpose and appropriate use of SMQs in safety surveillance activities.

The first edition of this report was published in 2004.[2] This second edition aims to include key information from the original edition and also to share the experience gained in the development and applications of SMQs since then.

The reader is referred to other useful tools that also provide guidance on the nature, development, and application of SMQs, including the *SMQ introductory guide*[3] produced by the MSSO and JMO for every new MedDRA version release. The reader may also wish to refer to the ICH-endorsed *MedDRA data retrieval and presentation: points to consider*[4] document for additional information. These resources are freely available from the MSSO at www.meddra.org. General training and information about MedDRA and SMQs is out of the scope of this publication, and interested individuals are advised to consult the ICH *Points to consider*[4] documents and the comprehensive training resources available from the MSSO and JMO.

I.C. Target audience

This publication is created to provide comprehensive information on the background, rationale and structure of SMQs for all who conduct analyses or reviews of data related to adverse effects of medical products. Specifically, it aims to inform individuals (including risk management physicians, pharmacoepidemiologists, toxicologists, statisticians, computer programmers, health informatics experts, medical writers and other interested parties) and groups in the following: biopharmaceutical industry; regulatory agencies; vendors of transactional safety databases and analytical tools; contract research organizations (CROs); independent advisory boards; data safety monitoring committees; poison control centres; medical device manufacturers; cosmetics industry; manufacturers of consumer health products; academic organizations; registries; hospitals and other interested organizations.

This report may also be used as a resource to promote awareness of the existence, utility and scope of SMQs.

References:

1. Introductory guide: MedDRA Version 18.0, MSSO-DI-6003-18.0.0, March 2015.
   See the relevant version on www.meddra.org
2. SMQs development and rational use of standardised MedDRA queries (SMQs). Retrieving adverse drug reactions with MedDRA. Report of the CIOMS Working Group. Geneva: CIOMS; 2004.
3. Introductory guide for Standardised MedDRA Queries (SMQs), Version 18.1, MSSO-DI-6226-18.1.0, September 2015.
   See the relevant version on www.meddra.org
4. MedDRA data retrieval and presentation: points to consider. ICH-endorsed guide for MedDRA users. Data output. Release 3.8, based on MedDRA version 17.1, September 2014.
   See the relevant version on www.meddra.org

CHAPTER II.
OVERVIEW OF SMQ CONCEPTS

Executive summary

SMQs are comprised of MedDRA PTs that focus on a defined medical condition. They are designed to assist in identifying and retrieving Individual Case Safety Reports (ICSR) that are potentially relevant to the condition of interest. Applying such standardised groups of terms as a supplement to the MedDRA hierarchy facilitates communication across organizations and over time. However, SMQs should not be expected to identify all relevant cases (i.e. some cases may be missed) and, indeed, an SMQ may identify some cases that are not relevant to the defined condition. Manual review of output is always appropriate. It should be noted that SMQs will not cover all topics that may be of interest to an organization; users may need to create their own ad hoc queries in these instances.

II.A. SMQ definition

SMQs are groupings of MedDRA PTs related to a defined medical condition or area of interest; they are intended to aid in the identification and retrieval of potentially relevant Individual Case Safety Reports. The terms in an SMQ may represent diagnoses, syndromes, symptoms, physical findings, procedures, laboratory and other physiological test data, all related to the condition or area of interest.

II.B. SMQ benefits and limitations

SMQs have several benefits to MedDRA subscribers and users. Most importantly, they are a standard tool to assist in the identification and retrieval of safety data and that facilitate comparison of safety data across products and in communications between organizations. As a standardised term list, an SMQ allows for a consistent data retrieval strategy that can be applied to many types of products, across organizations, and allow comparisons over time. Finally, the MSSO and JMO update SMQs with each new MedDRA version, relieving users of the resource burden associated with maintenance of reusable queries.

The limitations of SMQs also need to be kept in mind. SMQs should not be expected to identify all relevant cases (i.e. some cases may be missed) and they may identify some cases that are not relevant to the defined condition. SMQs do not, and are not ever expected to, cover all possible safety topics of interest to MedDRA subscribers; this means that a user may still need to create an ad hoc query when no SMQ of interest to the user exists. Ad hoc queries, by definition, should not be considered SMQs. In some cases, an ad hoc query may be found so useful that it can be submitted to the WG and MSSO for consideration as a topic of interest that may warrant development of a new SMQ (see Section II.D). Also, SMQs continue to evolve and change on the basis of maintenance activities, including real-world usage and subscriber change requests.

II.C. SMQ applications

SMQs aid in the retrieval of cases of interest by supplementing the MedDRA hierarchical structure in three ways:

- Importantly, the content of any given grouping term in MedDRA SOC (HLT or HLGT) may not be comprehensive for the condition/area of interest to the user. Thus, terms from multiple groupings are typically brought together within an SMQ.

- Terms in some MedDRA SOCs are not multiaxial (i.e. they are linked only to a single SOC by MedDRA placement rules). SMQs have collections of terms that are not subject to the restrictions of the placement rules for such terms in the MedDRA hierarchy (i.e. they can also contain terms from the SOC *Investigations*).

- SMQs are often developed to allow both a more *specific* search (i.e. to identify terms more likely to be associated with a condition, defined in a "narrow" search) as well as to allow a more *sensitive* search for all possible cases, including poorly described cases. The latter is a "broad" search that captures the majority of terms that might be associated with a condition. This structure allows the MedDRA subscriber to choose the most appropriate scope of the search to address the question of interest. See also "SMQ design features" in Section II.F for a detailed explanation.

As a practical approach when considering a data retrieval topic that is not easily satisfied using the basic MedDRA hierarchy, users are encouraged to first review the list of available SMQs (e.g. through a browser) and select one or more that would logically apply to the question being posed. Next, review of the documentation for the selected SMQ(s) in the *SMQ introductory guide*[1] of the respective MedDRA version is recommended as this will provide information on the definition and intent of the SMQ, as well as the expected query results. The definition of the concept that the SMQ was designed to address is particularly important. Finally, a MedDRA subscriber may wish to review the list of PTs of an SMQ to furthermore ensure that the terms relate to the medical condition or specific area of interest to the user.

After checking that the data to be searched are all coded with the same version of MedDRA and that the SMQ version matches the MedDRA version of the coded data, the selected SMQ can be used to identify potentially relevant Individual Case Safety Reports.

Safety assessors should understand that the raw results of an SMQ search may not be sufficient to directly address the question at hand. Application of the SMQ search is the first step in the assessment phase; completion of the task of retrieval of cases of interest using an SMQ involves review of the retrieved data. For example, the search results may contain cases that do not relate specifically to the condition/area of interest – i.e. these cases are noncontributory or represent "noise". Such results are usually to be expected when a broad search strategy is employed (see Section II.F).

Examples of settings in which SMQs may be useful are given below (note that the list may not be comprehensive and that there may be other potential uses for SMQs):

- analysis of aggregate safety data, including systematic reviews such as meta-analysis;[2]
- support for the preparation of medical quality review meetings and interim safety analyses;
- signal detection;
- monitoring of a potential safety risk (e.g. a known class effect);
- periodic reporting of aggregate data (e.g. DSUR, PSUR, Periodic Benefit–Risk Evaluation Report [PBRER]);
- tracking of important identified and important potential risks in risk management plans;
- as a focused search for medical review of cases/events of interest (e.g. responding to a regulatory enquiry); and
- single case/event alert – if supported by the safety system, SMQ terms can be employed in an automated notification to alert the assessor of a case/event needing immediate review.

Additional work has been done to explore application of SMQs in the regulatory decision-making process in areas such as safety signal detection, [3, 4] comparative risk of seizures, [5] influenza vaccine safety, [6] hepatobiliary disorders in Serbia, [7] and risk of depression or self-injury. [8]

II.D. Development of SMQs

One of the earliest tasks of the CIOMS SMQ WG was to create a list of potential topics that would be relevant candidates for query development. A list of approximately 100 concepts was developed, and these concepts formed the basis for the majority of SMQs in production at the time of this publication; other SMQ topic recommendations have been generated through a change request process administered by the MSSO and JMO.

Requests for new SMQs (or requests for revisions of previously published SMQs) that occur through the change request process are evaluated by an ICH Advisory Panel, a subgroup of members of the CIOMS SMQ WG who represent the ICH Parties. Users requesting a new or revised SMQ are asked to justify why there is a need for the proposed SMQ topic and also to describe potential alternatives to an SMQ. If, following evaluation of the responses to these questions, the ICH Advisory Panel endorses the request for a new SMQ, a CIOMS SMQ WG team is assembled to develop and test the SMQ content and structure (see Section II.F). The ICH Advisory Panel and the ICH MMB must approve any new SMQs before they are authorized for production – i.e. before being made available to MedDRA subscribers.

The definitions, inclusion and exclusion criteria, and descriptions of the hierarchy (if applicable) and algorithm (if applicable) for each SMQ are included in the *SMQ introductory guide,* [1] which is maintained by the MSSO and JMO and is available on their respective websites (www.meddra.org). The *SMQ introductory guide* [1] is part of each MedDRA subscriber's download package. Other supporting documentation for SMQs on the MSSO and JMO websites include:

- an SMQ spreadsheet (Excel format);
- information on the development status of proposed SMQs;
- SMQ original documentation from the CIOMS SMQ WG (includes details of testing for each SMQ in production);
- information about SMQ change requests and considerations for requests for new SMQs;
- information about rejected, suspended and discontinued SMQs;
- frequently asked questions about SMQs; and
- a version report (MedDRA Version Analysis Tool [MVAT]) that compares any two versions (e.g. the current and previous SMQ versions).

II.E. MedDRA Version Analysis Tool (MVAT)

The MedDRA Version Analysis Tool assists MedDRA subscribers by comparing and identifying changes between any two versions of MedDRA, including nonconsecutive versions. The tool can identify both "SMQ changes" and "PT changes within each SMQ", comparing two MedDRA releases both as a whole or only related to a specific set of MedDRA terms that the user may be interested in. This includes content changes described below.

As noted above, the term content of an SMQ consists of PTs. Terms representing the condition, characteristic and potential signs, symptoms, complications and related investigations are initially collected. Terms are selected for inclusion following a top-to-bottom and bottom-to-top search of the MedDRA hierarchy, as well as those from the *General disorders and administration site conditions, Social circumstances, Surgical and medical procedures,* etc. Each of the subordinate LLTs linked to the included PTs are also indirectly part of the SMQ; no LLT is included in an SMQ unless its parent PT is part of the SMQ also. In rare instances when an LLT has the desired specificity but is not represented as a unique concept at the PT level, the CIOMS SMQ IWG may request promotion of the term to a PT. If the change request is successful, the new PT is subsequently included in the SMQ. See Appendix 2 for additional information on term selection.

Every SMQ, and every PT included in an SMQ, has an assigned status of either "active" or "inactive":

▶ An active SMQ is included in the current version of MedDRA; an inactive SMQ is no longer maintained. An SMQ may be made inactive if it has been found to not be useful to users, becomes outdated, or is found to be otherwise problematic. An example of an inactivation is the SMQ *Adverse pregnancy outcome/reproductive toxicity (incl neonatal disorders)* which was made inactive due to problematic results in data retrieval after the SMQ had been released. This SMQ was substituted by the newly developed, more comprehensive and more clearly structured SMQ *Pregnancy and neonatal topics*.

PTs that have been made inactive in an SMQ are retained in their SMQ and are not deleted. An "inactive" status of a PT may be assigned if the term is found to have been included in error, if the inclusion criteria of the SMQ have changed, or if justified by changes in medical or regulatory science or due to restructuring of the SMQ. If an LLT is moved to a PT that is not part of the SMQ, it will also be made inactive. This concept of "inactive" is different from the concept of "non-current" as applied only to coding with LLTs. When applying an SMQ for data retrieval, inactive LLTs and PTs should be removed from the search.

II.F. SMQ design features

Once a topic of interest is approved for SMQ development, scientific consideration of the topic and subsequent test results are the main factors that inform selection of the best suited structure for the SMQ. Conceptually, the structures of SMQs have three basic design characteristics, as detailed below. Nearly all SMQs have both broad and narrow term groupings. Note that, while users may modify terms to customize a query, users do not have the option of changing the structural design features of a given SMQ – i.e. a narrow search that does not have an algorithmic feature cannot be converted to a narrow search with an algorithm.

SMQ structural design features are described as follows:

- ## II.F.i. Narrow/broad scope

This is the most common and fundamental feature of an SMQ. The term content for almost all SMQs consists of both narrow scope terms and broad scope terms. Some SMQs have only narrow scope terms. For example, SMQ *Taste and smell disorders* includes only narrow search terms, as there are not many nonspecific MedDRA PTs that describe these conditions. There are currently no MedDRA v18.0 SMQs with only broad terms.

The narrow scope terms of an SMQ are highly likely to represent the condition of interest and, therefore, confer specificity to the results of the search. In contrast, broad scope terms are less specific and may retrieve cases/events of interest but may also retrieve some data that are not cases/events of interest. However, broad terms confer sensitivity to the search results because of a lower chance of missing cases/events of interest. When performing a narrow search, only the narrow terms are used; when performing a broad search, narrow and broad terms (i.e. all the terms in the SMQ) are used (see Figure II.F.1).

Figure II.F.1. Depiction of two types of SMQ

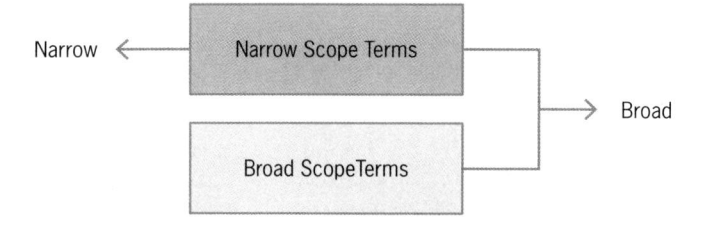

```
Narrow ← [Narrow Scope Terms] ┐
                              ├→ Broad
         [Broad ScopeTerms]   ┘
```

- ## II.F.ii. Hierarchical SMQs

Some SMQs are hierarchical – i.e. they are a set of queries related to one another in a hierarchical relationship. It is important to note that the hierarchical relationship between SMQs does not relate at all to the five-level hierarchy of terms in the MedDRA terminology. For SMQs, the hierarchy consists of one or more subordinate SMQs that are combined to create a superordinate, more inclusive SMQ. For example, the term content of the level-1 (top of the hierarchy) SMQ *Haematopoietic cytopenias* is formed by a combination of the term content of the four level-2 SMQs for *Haematopoietic erythropenia, Haematopoietic leukopenia, Haematopoietic thrombocytopenia*, and *Haematopoietic cytopenias affecting more than one blood cell type* (Figure II.F.2). Note that each of the four level-2 SMQs – such as SMQ *Haematopoietic erythropenia* – is also a stand-alone SMQ and can be used as such if the user wishes to retrieve only cases related to this particular form of cytopenia. Hierarchical SMQs can have as many as 5 levels, as for SMQ *Hepatic disorders*, or as few as 2 levels, as in the example of SMQ *Haematopoietic cytopenias*. Level-2 to level-5 SMQs are also referred to as sub-SMQs.

Figure II.F.2. Depiction of a hierarchical SMQ (MedDRA v18.0) *

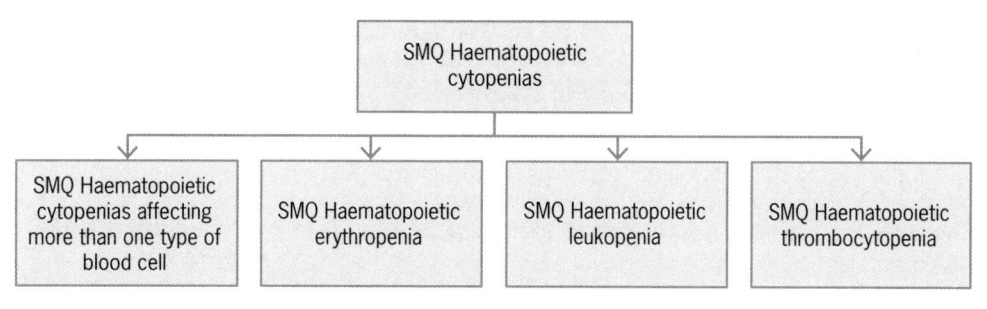

```
                    [SMQ Haematopoietic cytopenias]
         ┌──────────────┬──────────────┬──────────────┐
         ↓              ↓              ↓              ↓
[SMQ Haematopoietic  [SMQ Haematopoietic  [SMQ Haematopoietic  [SMQ Haematopoietic
 cytopenias affecting    erythropenia]        leukopenia]        thrombocytopenia]
 more than one type of
     blood cell]
```

* This figure is valid for the MedDRA version given, but please see also the current MedDRA/SMQ version.

- ## II.F.iii. Algorithmic SMQs

Some SMQs are designed to employ a stepwise (algorithmic) approach to the query. For these SMQs, the broad scope terms are further subdivided into categories of similar terms and designated as Category B, Category C and so on (narrow terms are always Category A for algorithmic SMQs). The theory behind an algorithmic SMQ is that a case is more likely to be of interest if it contains a defined *combination* of broad terms than if it contains any one broad term. The intention behind algorithmic designs is to reduce "noise" when applied to a large database. Algorithmic search methodology yields greater sensitivity compared to the narrow search and greater specificity compared to the broad search. An algorithmic approach is particularly helpful for those conditions of interest that are syndromes – i.e. constellations of signs and symptoms – such as SMQ *Anaphylactic reaction* or SMQ *Anticholinergic syndrome*. The categories and algorithms are unique and specific for each algorithmic SMQ. For example, categories B, C and D for SMQ *Anaphylactic reaction* are respiratory, skin/swelling and cardiovascular manifestations respectively, while those for SMQ *Anticholinergic syndrome* are nervous system, psychiatric and other anticholinergic syndrome manifestations respectively. The algorithms for cases of interest for each of these SMQs are also different (Table II.F.1).

Table II.F.1. Two examples of algorithmic SMQs *

SMQ *Anaphylactic reaction*	SMQ *Anticholinergic syndrome*
A or (B and C) or (D and (B or C))	A or (B and C and D)

* See also changes in the current SMQ version.

In the second example (SMQ *Anticholinergic syndrome*), a case is retrieved when it contains an event coded to the single PT of the narrow sub-SMQ or if it contains events that are coded to PTs from the broad categories B and C and D of this SMQ. Use of an algorithm is not required in order to be able to retrieve cases of interest using a particular SMQ. Application of the algorithm may be most helpful when it is expected that a large number of cases will be retrieved by broad scope terms; the algorithm may reduce the need for manual sorting of cases of interest. As of the time of the publication of this document, there is a single SMQ – SMQ *Systemic lupus erythematosus* – that employs a weighted algorithm. In this instance, each term in the eight different broad scope categories is assigned a "weight" ranging from 1 to 3. A case of interest is defined as one that contains a Category A (narrow) term or one with a set of broad terms whose combined "weight" total is equal to or greater than seven in this example.

II.G. SMQ modifications and organization-specific queries

One of the main purposes of using SMQs is to provide the user community with a standard tool to assist in the identification and retrieval of safety data. The existing SMQs provide a reasonable number of topics that are of interest for biopharmaceutical product safety surveillance and for surveillance of other medical products. The need for organization-developed queries may decline with each MedDRA version as additional SMQs are released and their range of topic coverage is extended. However, there will always be situations where SMQ modifications will be needed, and organizations may still need internal queries for topics not covered by existing SMQs.

Organization-developed queries should not be called "SMQs" even if the content and structure is similar to an SMQ. The *MedDRA data retrieval and presentation: points to consider*[9] document provides guidance on how to construct (and how to refer to) organization-specific queries for use on MedDRA-coded data. It is recommended that these "home-made" queries should be saved for future use and that detailed documentation should be maintained on the content, purpose, inclusion and exclusion criteria, the MedDRA version at the time, and other characteristics of these queries. For these customized queries, it is important to realize that maintenance is needed with each MedDRA release, and that the organization that created the query is responsible for its updating. It may be worthwhile to consider submitting a change request to the MSSO and JMO for a new SMQ if the proposed query may be useful to other MedDRA subscribers.

Similar to customized searches, any modification made to the term content or structure of an SMQ needs to be clearly stated to be transparent. A few SMQs are intended to be modified by the user depending on the compounds to which they are applied. For example, SMQ *Lack of efficacy/effect* is designed as a narrow search but contains only very nonspecific PTs that describe the failed effect of a drug in general terms. If the drug under study is, for example, an anti-asthmatic, then the SMQ could be amended by adding PTs for signs and symptoms of the lack of effect such as PT *Wheezing*, PT *Bronchospasm*, etc.

Such a modified SMQ should not be called a "SMQ" but should be referred to as a "modified MedDRA query based on an SMQ" and the referenced SMQ should be identified.

For other SMQs, the user may want to apply only part of the content (e.g. only the narrow terms or only one of several sublevels). All such applications of this kind are acceptable and valid as long as they are clearly documented (see Chapter V for additional details). For example, if a company wishes to identify all subjects who developed Systemic lupus erythematosus (SLE) after receiving a new medication, the SMQ *Systemic lupus erythematosus* may be used to query the safety database. Although systemic symptoms of SLE may include fever, the PT *Pyrexia* was not included in the SMQ *Systemic lupus erythematosus* (see the exclusion criteria for this SMQ, as described in the *SMQ introductory guide*[1]). The review of Individual Case Safety Reports often indicates that nonspecific terms such as pyrexia will likely identify several reports where the underlying reason for the fever was a common cold, a urinary tract infection or other etiologies other than SLE and hence may create noise. If a MedDRA subscriber considers to add potentially "noisy" terms to a modified MedDRA query based on an SMQ, such PTs should be included in the broad scope category.

II.H. SMQ maintenance

Once in production, SMQs are subject to the same change request process as other MedDRA change requests; they are considered simple change requests and are part of the permitted 100 requests per month per MedDRA subscriber. In addition to evaluating subscriber-initiated change requests along with the ICH Advisory Panel, the MSSO reviews all MedDRA term changes (e.g. new PTs, demotions, promotions, etc.) for potential impact on each SMQ in production.

Change requests for SMQs may result in (but are not limited to) the following:

- addition of PTs to an SMQ;
- change of the status of a PT from active to inactive (effectively removing a PT from current application of an SMQ);
- update of a term scope field of a PT (e.g. from broad to narrow or narrow to broad);
- update of an SMQ note – i.e. changes in the wording of the note field in the distributed ASCII file text;
- moving of an SMQ (e.g. change in the hierarchical position of an SMQ);
- addition of a new SMQ; or
- modifications to an SMQ name or SMQ documentation.

For a list of all SMQ change request actions, refer to Appendix B of the *MedDRA Change request information*[10] document. Approved SMQ changes are included in the MedDRA supplemental postings together with all other MedDRA changes and a summary is included in the *What's new*[11] document that is provided with each MedDRA version. In addition, a detailed listing of all term changes for the version is posted by the MSSO and JMO via an Excel spreadsheet. Information on specific changes which occurred since the release of the prior version is available in the version report. Retesting of SMQs on the basis of version-related changes is generally not part of the up-versioning process. However, in situations where changes may have significant impact on search results, the MSSO may ask the requesting subscriber to provide testing results, or they may consult the CIOMS SMQ WG about re-testing.

II.I. Consideration of requests for new SMQs

According to WHO, pharmacovigilance is defined as the science and activities relating to the detection, assessment, understanding and prevention of adverse effects or any other drug-related problem. This definition is also referenced in the *ICH E2E guideline*.[12] Pharmacovigilance is not a static process; thus, there is a need for continued development of new SMQs and refinement of existing SMQs to benefit the community of MedDRA subscribers. In May 2007 a process was implemented to accept new requests for SMQs through the MSSO/JMO change request process. Subscribers are asked to provide information to support each request via an electronic form which is available at the MedDRA website (www.meddra.org). This includes the intended application of the query, its general applicability, an explanation of why the existing MedDRA hierarchy is not suited to addressing the retrieval of cases of interest, and background information for the strategy that has been used thus far to identify cases of interest.

Requests for new SMQs are submitted to either the MSSO or JMO; the process for evaluation of requests has evolved with time and currently MSSO ensures that these requests are forwarded to the ICH Advisory Panel whose members review the request from the perspective of clinical relevancy and the potential for use by the broader community of MedDRA subscribers. The panel also evaluates the request in the context of the existing hierarchy and for potential overlap or possible synergy with SMQs already in production. After consideration of these points, the Panel will make a recommendation to the CIOMS SMQ IWG to proceed or not with development of the new SMQ.

If the panel recommends not proceeding, this decision and the rationale for it is provided to the requesting subscriber by the MSSO and JMO. This information is also noted in the general change request explanatory/rejection statements posted by MSSO and JMO. The requesting subscriber may provide additional explanatory documentation to support reconsideration of a rejected change request.

The change request process is also used for requests for modifications to existing SMQs, such as addition of a term.

More details regarding change requests for SMQs are available on the MedDRA website (www.meddra.org).

II.J. Testing of SMQs

Pre-release testing of SMQs provides a level of assurance that, when applied to real data, each candidate SMQ will identify a reasonable pool of ICSRs to be included in a case review for the medical condition or area of interest. Since the purpose of developing SMQs is to aid in ICSR retrieval, the purpose of pre-release testing does not extend to any estimate of either the predictive value positive or the predictive value negative of a given SMQ. Nevertheless, successful completion of testing for each candidate SMQ is required before that particular SMQ can be released to MedDRA subscribers.

- ### II.J.i. Historical background

The initial process for SMQ development used a two-phase testing approach in which the initial testing (Phase I) was coordinated by members of the CIOMS SMQ WG. For the second step in testing (Phase II), the MSSO in conjunction with the WG, made the candidate SMQ term list and draft documentation available to MedDRA subscribers to use with a request for subscriber feedback. The first SMQs were formally finalized and put into production after consideration of subscriber feedback from Phase II testing.

Subscriber feedback from Phase II testing was minimal. Thus, in July 2006 a decision was taken to remove Phase II testing from the SMQ development process to accelerate timely availability to subscribers. Currently, subscriber feedback is encouraged after an SMQ is released and in use by MedDRA subscribers. Any feedback received is treated as a MedDRA change request. The subscriber may be asked to provide more detail regarding their request, such as test results to support the request, and to ensure the changes would benefit the SMQ. After 18–24 months in production, the WG reviews each SMQ including changes to the SMQ that have occurred based on the routine maintenance process and subscriber feedback.

II.J.ii. Term list development

At the time of publication of this report, the MSSO does the initial research once a candidate SMQ is endorsed for development by the ICH Advisory Panel. This includes a proposal for the definition of the medical condition of interest and development of a draft term list; in some cases, the MSSO may propose revisions to a term list submitted by a subscriber as part of a request for a new SMQ. The medical literature and/or medical experts in the field of interest are consulted as needed when generating the candidate SMQ term list.

II.J.iii. Selection of SMQ development team

A team of several experts from the CIOMS SMQ WG is selected to complete the development and testing of the SMQ. The WG strives to include at least one regulator and one company database in the testing.

The team is responsible for:

- development of a workplan with milestones and timelines;
- review of the proposed definition and term lists for any additional concepts or PTs;
- determination of the need for expertise beyond the WG and securing this when needed;
- definition of criteria for acceptance or rejection of a candidate term;
- completion of testing of the term lists in their respective databases;
- analysis and summary of test results;
- discussion and communication as needed by e-mail/teleconferences/webinars;
- presentation of test results to the entire CIOMS SMQ WG at face-to-face meetings;
- based on input from the WG, completion of any additional steps or testing;
- after approval and acceptance of the candidate SMQ by the CIOMS SMQ WG, providing the MSSO with test results and background documentation; and
- assisting the MSSO when change requests are made.

II.J.iv. Testing parameters

All candidate SMQs are tested with data from pharmacovigilance databases. Ideally, testing is done in at least one regulatory database and one large company database with data on a variety of product exposures. In some cases, testing is also done in additional regulatory and/or company databases, since MedDRA coding conventions and practices may vary between institutions (e.g. number of terms per case, focus on diagnostic concepts vs. individual event terms, etc.).

The most common method of testing is to query the databases with the SMQ and specific products. Appropriate test products include those with the medical condition of interest listed in the regulator-approved product label information. In many cases testing is also done on products unlikely to be associated with the SMQ to evaluate the relative specificity of general terms. Another method used has been a general query of the database with the SMQ without selecting a specific product. In either case, the results of the queries are reviewed to verify whether or not the SMQ was successful in retrieving cases of interest, and to assess whether any changes to the structure of the SMQ are needed or if any additional terms should be added. In particular, the testing may provide a basis for allocating PTs to either narrow or broad searches. Retesting may be required, particularly in cases where additional test products need to be evaluated to determine the usefulness of selected PTs. The retesting will depend on the extent of revision recommended after initial testing.

II.K. Summary of concepts and proposals for use of SMQs

SMQs arose out of a recognized need of the MedDRA subscriber community for standard tools to assist in the identification and retrieval of safety data. They are developed by the CIOMS SMQ WG which is an ICH endorsed group of senior scientists from several regulatory authorities, international pharmaceutical companies, the MSSO, the JMO, WHO and other institutions.

At the time of the introduction of MedDRA v18.0, there were 98 SMQ topics (level-1 SMQs) available that contained a further 116 sub-SMQs within them (hierarchical SMQs).[B] SMQs have several benefits: they are a form of standardised communication that facilitates comparison of safety data across products and between organizations. As a standardised term list, an SMQ allows consistent data retrieval that can be applied over time and among many types of products. The MSSO and JMO update SMQs with each new MedDRA version, relieving subscribers of the maintenance burden associated with reusable queries.

Settings in which SMQs can be applied include the analysis of aggregate data and monitoring of a potential safety risk and for signal detection and responding to regulatory queries. They can also be used for safety assessment activities, including signal detection, periodic reporting, identification of cases/events for targeted assessment, and automated notification of single cases/events of interest.

The term content of an SMQ consists of MedDRA PTs. An "active" SMQ is one that is currently maintained by the MSSO. An "inactive" SMQ is no longer maintained. New SMQs can be requested by MedDRA subscribers through a change request process administered by the MSSO and JMO. If the ICH Advisory Panel approves the request, an SMQ WG team is formed to initiate the development of the SMQ.

SMQs do not, and are never expected to, cover all possible safety topics of interest to MedDRA subscribers; this means that a user may still need to create an ad hoc query when no SMQ of interest to the user exists. If any modifications are made to term content or structure of an SMQ by a subscriber or user, it can no longer be called a "SMQ" but it should instead be referred to as a "modified MedDRA query based on an SMQ".

SMQs continue to evolve and change based on maintenance activities, including real-world usage.

References:

1. Introductory guide for Standardised MedDRA Queries (SMQs), Version 18.1, MSSO-DI-6226-18.1.0, September 2015. See the relevant version on www.meddra.org
2. Gopal S, Hough D, Karcher K, Nuamah I, Palumbo J, Berlin JA, et al. Risk of cardiovascular morbidity with risperidone or paliperidone treatment: analysis of 64 randomized, double-blind trials. J Clin Psychopharmacol. 2013; 33(2):157–61.
3. Newbould V, Halsey N, Tsintis P, Lerch M, Mozzicato P. Standardised MedDRA queries: Analysis of their signal detection capability. 22nd International Conference on Pharmacoepidemiology, Lisbon, 24-27 August 2006: Abstract 87.
4. Berlin C, Blanch C, Lewis DJ, Maladorno DD, Michel C, Petrin M, et al. Are all quantitative postmarketing signal detection methods equal? Performance characteristics of logistic regression and multi-item gamma Poisson Shrinker. Pharmacoepidemiol Drug Saf. 2012; Jun 21(6):622–30. doi: 10.1002/pds.2247. Epub 2011 Oct 12.
5. Lertxundi U, Hernandez R, Medrano J, Domingo-Echaburu S, Garcıa M, Aguirre C. Antipsychotics and seizures: higher risk with atypicals? Seizure. 2013; 22(2):141–3. doi: 10.1016/j.seizure.2012.10.009. Epub 2012 Nov 10.
6. Vellozzi C, Broder KR, Haber P, Guh A, Nguyen M, Cano M, et al. Adverse events following influenza A (H1N1) 2009 monovalent vaccines reported to the vaccine adverse event reporting system, United States, October 1, 2009–January 31, 2010. Vaccine. 2010; 28(45):7248–55.
7. Petronijevic M, Ilic K, Suzuki A. Drug induced hepatotoxicity: data from the Serbian pharmacovigilance database. Pharmacoepidemiol Drug Saf. 2011; 20:416–23.
8. Moore TJ, Furberg CD, Glenmullen J, Maltsberger JT, Singh S. Suicidal behavior and depression in smoking cessation treatments. PLoS ONE. 2011; Nov 2;6(11):e27016.
9. MedDRA data retrieval and presentation: points to consider. ICH-endorsed guide for MedDRA users on data output. Release 3.8, based on MedDRA version 17.1, September 2014. See the relevant version on www.meddra.org
10. MedDRA Change request information. MSSO-DI-6282-3.3.0, 2 April 2015. See the relevant version on www.meddra.org
11. MedDRA What's new. MedDRA v18.1, MSSO-DI-6001-18.1.0, September 2015. See the relevant version on www.meddra.org
12. ICH E2E guideline. Harmonised tripartite guideline pharmacovigilance planning. Current Step 4 version, 18 November 2004. Geneva: International Conference on Harmonisation; 2004.

[B] Note that these numbers will adjust over time with new MedDRA versions.

CHAPTER III.

SEARCH STRATEGIES WITH A FOCUS ON PHARMACOVIGILANCE

Executive summary

SMQs can be used in routine pharmacovigilance activities to enhance the quality and reproducibility of analyses across the entire life cycle of a medicinal product. The full scope of a search (also called "broad SMQ" or "broad search")[C] – i.e. the combination of both broad and narrow scope terms of an SMQ – should be used when maximum sensitivity of a search is required. However, this broad search may retrieve cases that are not relevant to the specific condition. Conversely, a narrow scope SMQ – i.e. only the narrow scope terms or the application of an algorithm, when one exists for the SMQ – may be used to increase specificity of the search, with the recognition that some relevant cases may not be identified. Additionally, some SMQs have a hierarchical layout (e.g. they consist of one or more subordinate SMQs that are combined to create a superordinate, more inclusive SMQ).

Many factors affect the quality of output obtained by applying an SMQ to a MedDRA-coded database. These factors, together with the purpose of the query, must be identified and considered when interpreting the results.

III.A. Introduction

This chapter reviews some of the advantages of using SMQs in conducting routine drug safety activities to enhance the quality and completeness of safety analyses. SMQs can be applied throughout the life cycle of a product to help provide a meaningful adverse reaction profile, to contribute to a comprehensive benefit–risk evaluation and for the early detection and evaluation of emerging safety signals. In general, it is recommended that SMQs are used unaltered – i.e. PT content of the SMQ should not be altered. Exclusion and inclusion criteria that were applied for term selection in defining the SMQ should be considered. To ensure that the search strategy is appropriate for the question, it is necessary to determine the nature of the safety topic and the purpose of the query. Almost all SMQs consist of both narrow scope terms and broad scope terms. The narrow scope terms of an SMQ are highly likely to represent the medical condition of interest and therefore confer specificity to the results of the search. One may apply a narrow SMQ to estimate the number of events/cases for a condition in order to decide whether a more complete search and review should be carried out. In contrast, broad scope terms are less specific (they often include nonspecific signs, symptoms and investigational findings that may represent the medical condition even in the absence of a diagnosis) and may lead to the retrieval of other conditions with different etiologies, thus decreasing specificity, but confer sensitivity to the search results because of a lower chance of missing cases/events of interest. An extensive search that includes a broad scope SMQ may be more appropriate for a regulatory query or evaluation of an emerging safety signal. In other instances, a combination of sub-SMQs (e.g. combination of several level-2 SMQs of a hierarchical SMQ) may be most appropriate. Examples are provided below to illustrate when the use of each of the above may be appropriate.

[C] Broad search and broad SMQ are used synonymously throughout this document.

When the intention of searching a database is to retrieve all possible cases of a medical concept, it is recommended that the full (i.e. broad) scope search is utilized, which includes both the "narrow" scope terms (specific to the medical condition) and the "broad" scope terms (often of a less specific nature). For example, SMQ *Dementia* has both narrow and broad scope terms; the narrow scope terms are specific to dementia (e.g. PT *Dementia*, PT *Dementia Alzheimer's type*, PT *Vascular dementia*, etc.), while the broad scope terms represent signs and symptoms that occur in dementia but are not specific only to this condition (e.g. PT *Memory impairment*, PT *Agnosia*, PT *Aphasia*, etc.). If the objective of a search is to review all potential cases of dementia in a treated population, both narrow and broad search terms from SMQ *Dementia* should be utilized to maximize sensitivity, since the signs and symptoms of dementia can be nonspecific. On the other hand, if the purpose of a search is to identify only cases that are highly likely to represent the condition of interest (i.e. if a greater specificity is needed) then it is appropriate to use a narrow SMQ (e.g. narrow scope terms of SMQ *Dementia*).

A combination of sub-SMQs can be used to identify relevant cases for a general concept. For example, to review cases of supraventricular tachyarrhythmia in an adult population, several sub-SMQs related to cardiac arrhythmias are depicted in Figure III.A.1.

Figure III.A.1. Hierarchical structure of SMQ *Cardiac arrhythmias*[D] (MedDRA v18.0) *

- SMQ Cardiac arrhythmias (SMQ)
    - SMQ Arrhythmia related investigations, signs and symptoms (SMQ)
    - SMQ Cardiac arrhythmia terms (incl bradyarrhythmias and tachyarrhythmias) (SMQ)
        - SMQ Bradyarrhythmias (incl conduction defects and disorders of sinus node fonction) (SMQ)
            - SMQ Bradyarrhythmia terms, nonspecific (SMQ)
            - SMQ Conduction defects (SMQ)
            - SMQ Disorders of sinus node function (SMQ)
        - SMQ Cardiac arrhythmia terms, nonspecific (SMQ)
        - SMQ Tachyarrhythmias (incl supraventricular and ventricular tachyarrhythmias) (SMQ)
            - SMQ Supraventricular tachyarrhythmias (SMQ)
            - SMQ Tachyarrhythmia terms, nonspecific (SMQ)
            - SMQ Ventricular tachyarrhythmias (SMQ)
    - SMQ Congenital and neonatal arrhythmias (SMQ)

* This figure is valid for the MedDRA version given, but please see also the current MedDRA/SMQ version.

For this particular search, it would be reasonable to exclude sub-SMQs that specifically retrieve bradyarrhythmias and congenital and neonatal arrhythmias. Also, depending on the objective of the search, one can further include or exclude nonspecific SMQs, such as SMQ *Tachyarrhythmia terms, nonspecific*.

The required specificity/sensitivity of the search drives the decision to utilize the narrow or broad scope terms of the included sub-SMQs. Any sub-SMQ may be used, if the title, definition and content match the objective of the search. However, to maintain the integrity of the referenced SMQ, the PT content of the SMQ should not be altered in any way; this applies to both terms and their associated scope (however see Sections II.G. and III.E. for additional guidance).

[D] The formats expressed as "SMQ *Cardiac arrhythmias*" and "*Cardiac arrhythmias* (SMQ)" are used interchangeably throughout this document.

III.B. General considerations for search strategies

• III.B.i. Factors which affect the quality of database queries

Completeness and accuracy of case reports

The completeness and accuracy of cases retrieved by a search are highly dependent upon the origin of the cases. Data from clinical trials, if careful analysis of event data is planned, can be very informative. For example, training clinical investigators in the reporting of safety/adverse events helps to provide high-quality initial data in natural language for ongoing medical monitoring of safety during a high-morbidity study. It also minimizes the need for subsequent data clarification. Ensuring that reports are complete and accurate prior to study database closure not only provides a quality study report in real time, but also stands in good stead later if the data are required for a regulatory submission or meta-analysis. It is usually not possible to clarify old data as the investigators of old clinical studies may no longer be contactable or the relevant records may not be available.

ICSRs reported spontaneously tend to be less complete than clinical trial reports and their content is often influenced by the type of reporter (consumer or health-care professional). If needed, it is advisable to request any clarification as soon as possible to minimize the risk of losing contact with the reporter or access to the relevant medical records.

Coding practices

The *MedDRA term selection: points to consider*[1] document is a global, ICH-endorsed guide for MedDRA subscribers to promote accurate and consistent term selection. Organizations are advised to base their coding practices on this document as closely as possible. However, the accuracy and consistency of coding within the same company may have changed over time with working practices, training, or even with product lines or technical capabilities of utilized tools. In the case of a merger, legacy data from two previously separate business entities are likely to have been coded differently and may have been up-versioned by applying different methods. Indeed, migration or recoding of pre-MedDRA data may have been from a verbatim term or directly from a coded term selected from a classification scheme with lesser specificity than MedDRA. More recent data within the newly formed company may follow different coding practices.

Specificity of the coding terminology

MedDRA was adopted by one regulatory authority in November 1997 and many organizations have subsequently implemented it on individual schedules. Part of MedDRA implementation entails conversion of pre-existing data coded in other terminologies. This may be particularly relevant for companies with a portfolio of well-established products, i.e. generic products that may have legacy data coded with terminologies in use prior to MedDRA adoption. In all such cases, the data migration method should be taken into account. If data migration utilized only the codes from the previous terminology, then the level of specificity remains unchanged, reflecting that of the terminology originally used to code those data. If the verbatim text from pre-existing data is recoded directly into MedDRA, it will bear the specificity of MedDRA and better match newly acquired data.

• III.B.ii. SMQs enhance the quality and efficiency of pharmacovigilance and promote harmonisation

Quality
- ensures search strategies are science-based, consistent, reproducible and complete, thus adding credibility to analysis results (standard and proven methodology). This in turn reduces bias in data outputs and facilitates standardised case identification processes;

- promotes meaningful comparison of current and previous safety profile;
- eliminates dependency on groups or individuals within one organization that may change during the course of the product life cycle;
- reduces the likelihood that external reviewers will draw different conclusions from source data; and
- enhances the quality of benefit–risk assessment.

Quality is dependent on accurate medical coding.

Efficiency
- simplifies up-versioning activities (replaces in-house searches that need to be maintained and provides more focused, standard search strategies); and
- streamlines the process of creating new search strategies where an SMQ is not available. If there is no suitable SMQ, the established method of creating SMQs discussed in prior sections of this book and the guidance provided in the *MedDRA data retrieval and presentation: points to consider*[2] document on how to construct (and how to refer to) organization-specific queries for use on MedDRA-coded data can be utilized in-house to create an ad hoc search strategy (this also facilitates a better match if an SMQ is subsequently created for that event of interest);

Harmonisation
- enhances standardisation of reference safety documents across an organization;
- enhances consistency of search strategies used across products;
- facilitates comparison of the safety profile of similar products;
- fosters early cross-functional cooperation – i.e. SMQs may be applied to clinical trial safety data as well as post-marketing data;
- provides a global standard and transparency in search strategies across all organizations using MedDRA-coded data.

• III.B.iii. Selection of an appropriate SMQ

Knowledge of the database and coding practices is required and it is necessary to be aware of changes in the database over time. Specific database fields (e.g. tick boxes, age range, etc.) may exist in addition to MedDRA coding. For example, the occurrence of pregnancy may be captured in a data field (tick box) in one database but another database may require the application of appropriate MedDRA codes. Both medical and technical expertise should be consulted to gain an understanding of the present database and practices as well as historical aspects.

It is recommended that the SMQ/list of MedDRA terms employed in a database search to identify, review and analyse cases of interest should be prespecified.

The reader may also wish to refer to the ICH-endorsed *MedDRA data retrieval and presentation: points to consider*[2] document for additional information. The document is updated periodically to remain consistent with releases of new versions of MedDRA.

After reviewing the *Introductory guide for standardised MedDRA queries*[3] that matches the MedDRA version for the dataset, one decides whether to apply the narrow or broad SMQ or, if the SMQ is hierarchical, one selects the appropriate part of the hierarchy or a combination of sub-SMQs. Narrow scope terms are used when a high specificity of the search is required (e.g. when the mechanism of action for a specific drug leads to expected event types). The broad scope search terms should be used when greater sensitivity is required (e.g. an initial evaluation of a condition for which the impact of the suspect medication is uncertain, such as immune disorders). On the other hand, in the case of syndromes (e.g. when a reported diagnosis is made based on a constellation of nonspecific clinical signs and symptoms), an algorithmic approach is particularly helpful (e.g. SMQ *Anaphylactic reaction*, and SMQ *Anticholinergic syndrome*). For those combined with a laboratory confirmation, as in the case of Creutzfeldt-Jacob disease, the nonspecific signs and symptoms *alone* may not efficiently identify cases of interest, but laboratory confirmation is required to make an accurate diagnosis. Algorithmic SMQs are intended for situations where application of the broad search terms tends to retrieve a large number of reports that, upon review, may prove not to represent cases of interest (i.e. "noise"). The application of the algorithm increases specificity and reduces "noise", thus generally limiting the need for manual sorting for cases of interest. For safety databases that are not able to automate the algorithm, it may be necessary to apply the algorithm manually after obtaining the initial output from the safety database. Additional technical details are provided in Chapter IV; considerations for use of algorithmic SMQs regarding dates of events are discussed below in Section III.D. To decide on the most appropriate scope of a search (degree of sensitivity and specificity), it is necessary to consider the product and background patient population. Some events may be due to the intended therapeutic use of the product and commonly reported, such as hypotension with beta blockers or cardiovascular events in the elderly. It may be necessary to consider subsets of data by dose if the product has a narrow therapeutic margin. One should also be aware of manifestations of the disease being treated or risk factors (e.g. renal impaired patients or the elderly).

III.C. Communication and documentation of the search strategy

The SMQ/MedDRA terms should be described in the appropriate sections of the respective documents (e.g. statistical analysis plans, signal detection strategies, risk management plans, clinical study reports, periodic reports, investigator brochures, labelling documents, etc.). Any regional regulatory templates or specific requirements should be borne in mind. Formal documentation of search strategy, including strengths and limitations of the dataset, is necessary for appropriate interpretation of the output. It is also necessary to communicate how the search was carried out and, when tracking an ongoing safety issue, the documentation should enable the search to be repeated at a future time.

The methodology used to identify cases of interest as well as any further steps/criteria to rule out specific cases or groups of adverse events should be described in the documents where the results are reported. The report should specify the type of search (e.g. narrow or broad search, algorithm, or combination of sub-searches of a hierarchical SMQ) used and the associated rationale (see Appendix 3, Table A.3.1).

- ### III.C.i. SMQ application considerations, interpretation of output

How/purpose

SMQs provide a standardised way to search pharmacovigilance databases. Their use is recommended by many regulators as a first search strategy to retrieve potential cases of interest. As SMQs are maintained centrally, regulatory authorities and industry will apply the same MedDRA PTs for a given version of MedDRA, as long as the SMQs have not been customized.

The output of an SMQ search is not, per se, the final dataset, neither does it constitute the safety profile for a product, nor does it imply causality between a suspect drug and the condition of interest. Further medical review is always needed to filter out "noise" (e.g. cases that, upon review, prove not to be of interest). Narrow searches are less likely to generate noise than broad searches. However, both should be considered when conducting thorough safety reviews.

Once the results from the SMQ search in a database become available, one may apply prespecified secondary definition criteria to the data.

Additionally, when investigating a signal, use of an SMQ rather than a single PT may add to the completeness of the search by retrieving cases that represent the condition of interest but may have been coded with a different PT. For example, SMQ *Torsade de pointes/QT prolongation* may retrieve cases of interest that would be missed if only PT *Torsade de pointes* was used.

For instance, if the narrow terms from SMQ *Hypersensitivity* are used to identify potential cases of infusion reaction, it is appropriate to further narrow down the results to cases where the adverse event occurred within 24 hours of suspect product infusion.

The results of an analysis with an SMQ can be further stratified by sex, time to onset of event, and other relevant factors. One may also predefine manual review criteria to facilitate by-pass of noncontributory cases from subsequent results (for instance, on the basis of biological implausibility or confounding factors that are prespecified in study reports).

Standardised searches can also be used to identify similar cases from different geographical areas, disease states, or subpopulations. In addition, the results contribute to understanding the safety profile for a medical product.

- ## III.C.ii. Signal detection

Traditional signal detection activities may be supported by data-mining tools that apply statistical methods with predefined thresholds to detect (e.g. an increase in frequency or reporting proportions of a specific event or disproportionality in reporting). For instance, a disproportionality may be observed when an event is reported more often for a specific product as compared with other products in the database (often the total of all other products is used, but also a subgroup or a specific product may be used). In order to detect an increase in reporting frequency/rate of a specific event, the reporting frequency/rate of this event in a predefined time period is compared with prior time periods. In both situations (disproportionality and increased reporting frequency), the user is alerted whenever the predefined threshold is reached.

Some signal detection tools are capable of applying SMQs in addition to single PTs. Using a group of specific PTs to define the adverse event of interest (e.g. narrow SMQ) might result in reaching the predefined threshold for a statistical method earlier than a single PT. However, there is also evidence for the opposite – i.e. the threshold for disproportionality might be reached earlier at PT level than at SMQ level.[4] Indeed, use of a broad scope might dilute a signal (i.e. reduce prominence of a disproportionality statistic). There is no uniform agreement on these points.

These statistical methods can also aid in identification of serious adverse event reports of interest and results can be further stratified – i.e. to screen for designated medical events, for review and expedited reporting where appropriate.

- ## III.C.iii. Risk management

Narrow SMQs may be applied to post-marketing data at intervals to track reporting rates of an event of interest. This is far more convenient and consistent than maintaining customized in-house searches. Regulatory authorities may be able to apply such screens to data from products of the same class. Further, actions may be necessary by Independent Data Monitoring Committees (IDMCs)/Data Safety Monitoring Boards (DSMBs) or the sponsor to manage risk when a prespecified threshold of an event of interest is reached. This applies to the analysis of safety data from clinical trials too.

- ## III.C.iv. Periodic safety reporting

SMQs should always be considered when generating searches for periodic reporting (e.g. PBRERs, PSURs, DSURs). For instance, the redesigned SMQ *Pregnancy and neonatal topics* facilitates the retrieval of pregnancy cases, especially if there is no database field available to identify such ICSRs directly.

Use of SMQs also enhances appropriate comparisons of reporting rates of conditions of interest over time. SMQs avoid the need for updates of company-specific selection of terms over time, and increase transparency, as well as comparability over time for one compound, or across multiple compounds. In the context of periodic safety reporting, using a narrow-scope SMQ may be considered more adequate since this would enhance specificity. The risk characteristics of the compound/product always need to be considered as well – i.e. clearly defined medical concepts vs. signs and symptoms which can have different diagnoses. It is essential to also consider in-house features such as database fields as well as coded MedDRA terms for completeness.

- ### III.C.v. Where to use SMQs (types of databases)

SMQs can be applied throughout the life cycle of a product, from interventional clinical trials to post-marketing data collected from spontaneous reporting. This adds consistency and validity to adverse event profiles associated with the product over time. Apart from searches carried out for reviews of an event of interest, SMQs may be imported into an active surveillance system to provide automated alerts for incoming cases that are likely to be the event being monitored. Dependent on the specificity of the SMQ or sub-SMQ, the narrow-scope query may be more suited to this type of safety surveillance system as use of the broad scope may introduce an unnecessary level of "noise".

It is conceptually useful for various end-users, including those who do not directly work with MedDRA-coded data, to be aware of the terms in SMQs and their content parameters (i.e. narrow or broad scope). For example, epidemiology data or data used for active safety surveillance are often from claims data or electronic health records, which are largely not coded in MedDRA. Also, in contrast to traditional pharmacovigilance databases, these data sources may have wide variations from country to country and in different health-care systems. Nevertheless, the availability and structure of SMQs may serve as a very useful conceptual approach for pharmacoepidemiologists to create analogous condition-based groupings of International Classification of Diseases (ICD) codes, for instance, and apply similar data retrieval strategies. Although the MedDRA codes are much more geared to describing clinical signs and symptoms, as compared to ICD codes that describe specific disorders (and less frequently include signs and symptoms) a similar effort for the use of ICD code grouping would be useful. In the future, there are likely to be crosswalk mappings between some MedDRA terms and terminologies used in pharmacoepidemiological databases; once these are in place, there may be opportunities to use SMQs directly to study these data. However, the appropriateness of applying queries to data sources used in non-interventional studies and active safety surveillance must be carefully considered in relation to aspects other than coding, particularly with respect to potential confounders and biases that could influence the results returned by a query.

- ### III.C.vi. Actual use in regulatory settings

This section contains descriptions of SMQ applications in the regulatory setting, including:

▶ lessons learned from implementation experience; and
▶ lessons learned in practical applications.

SMQs are used by regulators, industry and academia to facilitate analysis of MedDRA-coded data, including detection and evaluation of safety signals. Since the SMQs are a standardised search tool, the results are more comparable than if SMQs are not used.

Regulatory agencies that have implemented MedDRA have also integrated SMQs into their internal search processes, automated tool functions and training curricula. Various other strategies may be applied, depending on the topic of concern and the character of the data and data sources, but the grouping of safety data by MedDRA hierarchy and by SMQs is a basic, initial, routine approach that has been widely adopted.

For example, both MedDRA hierarchy groupings and SMQs are routinely used in exploratory analysis of clinical trial data to view possible disparity between comparator groups and to focus further review.

SMQs are also routinely applied to post-marketing data to aid in identifying or characterizing safety signals. Also, regulatory authorities often request that a sponsor employ one or more SMQs so that data can be reported and reviewed in that context and in a standardised manner.

Cases identified by the application of an SMQ should always be reviewed for relevance.

- ### III.C.vii. Monitoring frequency of events in clinical trials or reporting rates for labelling

SMQs may be used to calculate the frequencies of adverse events reported in clinical trials, thus contributing to the establishment of the safety profile of an authorized product in labelling documents. Instead of manually selecting different PTs for an expected adverse event, an SMQ averts the need for continuous updates of hand-picked terms throughout the development programme and increases comparability between different studies in the same programme as well as with compounds of the same class in a harmonised way.

The same applies to the life cycle of a marketed product for which trials and label updates are performed. When using SMQs in this context, one has to bear in mind the different scopes (narrow vs. broad), hierarchical and algorithmic possibilities. In other words, for labelling and signal detection purposes, a narrow/specific approach might be considered more adequate, compared to applying a broad/sensitive search to activities such as signal evaluation. Consideration must also be given to the risk characteristics of the compound/product – i.e. clearly defined medical concepts vs. signs and symptoms that may be common to several different diagnoses.

It is very important, particularly when analysing post-marketing data, to highlight the pitfalls when an estimated denominator has a high degree of uncertainty. However, SMQs applicable for events of interest may be applied to clinical trial monitoring of incoming reports of adverse events where the denominator is defined to a greater degree. Although this may be blinded data, events of interest identified by the narrow SMQ facilitate medical review and rapid follow-up of reports for more details. SMQs may also facilitate the gathering of data provided to IDMC/DSMB and support medical quality review meetings for clinical trials.

Many organizations monitor medically important safety data that can have an impact on the benefit–risk evaluation of a product with or without public health implications. When monitoring for such events, SMQs containing a cluster of specific PTs can provide greater sensitivity relative to a single PT describing the event of interest. For instance, Stevens-Johnson syndrome could be detected with greater sensitivity by the narrow search of SMQ *Severe cutaneous adverse reaction* compared to a search using only the single PT *Stevens-Johnson syndrome*. Similarly, the designated medical event "bone marrow failure" could be detected by SMQ *Agranulocytosis* and SMQ *Haematopoietic cytopenias*. Depending on the type of disorder being queried, one may choose to include the appropriate SMQ/sub-SMQ that meets the objective of the question. For example, haematopoietic cytopenias affecting more than one type of blood cell are comprised of these sub-SMQs: SMQ *Haematopoietic erythropenia*, SMQ *Haematopoietic leukopenia* and SMQ *Haematopoietic thrombocytopenia*. One may choose to employ one, all or any combination of the three sub-SMQs to respond to an internal or external data enquiry.

III.D. Limitations – guidelines to avoid pitfalls

Familiarity with the *Introductory guide for standardised MedDRA queries*[3] for the relevant SMQ is necessary – particularly the definition of the condition of interest and the inclusion and exclusion criteria that underlie the choice of SMQ design. One should consider the inclusion and exclusion criteria for the search strategy to ensure that the SMQ meets one's intended needs.

However, if the SMQ does not meet the need, it may be necessary to customize the query (see Section III.E). The inclusion and exclusion criteria should also be considered when reviewing and interpreting data retrieved by the search strategy.

For certain SMQs the list of PTs is limited to a core set of terms as not all possible signs and symptoms can be captured that may be applicable to every product. For example, the SMQ *Lack of efficacy/effect* consists only of a narrow search, which contains a list of PTs applicable to a large number of compounds. The user may, however, add PTs to the search strategy by taking into consideration the type of product and/or indication (e.g. signs and symptoms of impaired glucose tolerance, etc.) for an antidiabetic product. See also Chapter II.

It may be necessary to conduct further searches using database fields or additional terms that would be appropriate for the product in question. For instance, a drug that has been marketed for over 20 years may record myocardial damage with laboratory tests predating the use of troponin or creatine phosphokinase-MB (both of which are in SMQ *Ischaemic heart disease*). The further search may include PTs reflecting the older tests of aspartate aminotransferase (AST) and lactate dehydrogenase (LDH). However, it is also possible that these latter terms may also generate a lot of "noise".

Safety profiling requires the contribution of many factors, and not just SMQs. The data retrieved from applying an SMQ must undergo medical review as there will inevitably be cases retrieved that prove not to be of interest, even after applying only the narrow search. For instance, mere use of a constrained list of terms cannot discriminate between ICSRs that are appropriately coded with those terms and ICSRs that do not fit the description of the event of interest but are coded as such. Furthermore, the timing of an event relative to the use of the product is not taken into account when applying an SMQ, so retrieved data will require review for plausible temporal relationships.

An important consideration when using algorithmic SMQs is that an algorithm is not affected by the dates of occurrence of the events. Thus the adverse events retrieved through the algorithm may have occurred at different time points without a temporal relation to each other. For example, using the algorithmic SMQ *Acute pancreatitis*, A or B+C would identify potential cases of acute pancreatitis for review. The PT *Amylase increased* is in category B and PT *Abdominal pain* is in category C. However, the algorithm will retrieve or identify cases where abdominal pain co-occurs with the increase in amylase, and cases where abdominal pain has an end-date many months prior to the event start-date of increased amylase. Therefore, additional data stratification may be needed to identify cases with events which are likely to have a temporal association (i.e. that occurred within an appropriate time interval).

For example, one may wish to apply further criteria to identify events that occurred within one week, or other appropriate time interval depending on the disease state or population, etc.

Furthermore, there are some SMQs, such as the SMQ *Demyelination*, where selected terms were excluded based on the results of pre-release testing. However, a user may wish to include such terms in a search to retrieve a comprehensive dataset if deemed appropriate in this situation. Such situations are addressed in the *Introductory guide for standardised MedDRA queries*,[3] as illustrated by the example of the SMQ *Demyelination*, where the following note is provided: "If searching for a de novo signal of demyelination, it is recommended to use the narrow and broad terms in this SMQ and also SMQ *Peripheral neuropathy* and SMQ *Guillain-Barre syndrome*. Broad terms for signs and symptoms of demyelinating diseases were excluded because they are in SMQ *Peripheral neuropathy* and SMQ *Guillain-Barre syndrome*. Some broad terms were also excluded as being too nonspecific, related to advanced demyelination, or because of poor performance in SMQ testing." The *SMQ introductory guide*[3] also notes that these excluded terms (see Tables III.D.1 and III.D.2) may be included in a search at the user's discretion, as long as this is clearly documented in the methodology section of the SMQ report.

Table III.D.1. Broad terms excluded because they are in the SMQs *Peripheral neuropathy* and/or *Guillain-Barre syndrome* (MedDRA v10.1) *

Areflexia	Neuropathy
Asthenia	Neuropathy peripheral
Balance disorder	Ophthalmoplegia

Coordination abnormal	Paraesthesia
Dysaesthesia	Paralysis
Dysphagia	Paralysis flaccid
Facial paresis	Peroneal nerve palsy
Gait disturbance	Quadriparesis
Hypoaesthesia	Sensory disturbance
Hyporeflexia	Sensory loss
Muscle atrophy	Speech disorder
Muscular weakness	Tremor

* See also changes in the current SMQ version.

Table III.D.2. Broad terms excluded because they are nonspecific, related to advanced demyelination, or did not test well during SMQ development (MedDRA v10.1) *

Abdominal discomfort	Nuclear magnetic resonance imaging abnormal
Back pain	Nystagmus (tested & found to be nonspecific)
Bowel incontinence	Pain
Confusional state	Pain in extremity
Constipation	Radial nerve palsy
Diplopia	Sexual dysfunction
Dizziness	Tremor
Fatigue	Urinary incontinence
Incontinence	Urinary retention
Mental status changes	Vertigo
Muscle spasms	Visceral pain
Muscle spasticity	Vision blurred
Musculoskeletal stiffness	Visual disturbance

* See also changes in the current SMQ version.

Another example is provided by the SMQ *Neuroleptic malignant syndrome.*

The term *Pyrexia* is included under the broad scope, hence a search of any large database using this SMQ will most likely identify a large number of cases of pyrexia, most often due to a common cold. However, in the absence of muscle rigidity, autonomic instability and cognitive changes, pyrexia alone is unlikely to identify true cases of neuroleptic malignant syndrome. Yet to maintain the standardised integrity of the SMQ, it is recommended that the full content, including PT *Pyrexia*, be applied as an initial step and appended to safety query reports for transparency. However, upon review of the results, pyrexia may be deemed too nonspecific to identify cases of neuroleptic malignant syndrome and, after describing the rationale in the query report, it is appropriate to indicate that such cases will not be discussed further in the query report.

The same MedDRA version for the SMQ and coded dataset must be used to ensure that query results are valid and to avoid data output errors because of potential differences in term placement in two or more different MedDRA versions. The ICH *MedDRA data retrieval and presentation: points to consider*[2] document provides an example of undesired consequences when the SMQ applied and the MedDRA-coded data in the database are of different MedDRA versions.

When repeating searches after a period of time, consider that some of the SMQs released with earlier MedDRA versions have been redesigned following user comments. The most marked example was SMQ *Adverse pregnancy outcome/reproductive toxicity (incl neonatal disorders)*. The initial form of this SMQ was not helpful in producing useful searches for PSURs. In response to user requests, this SMQ was made inactive (as described in Section II.E of MedDRA Version Analysis Tool [MVAT]). A new, redesigned SMQ – SMQ *Pregnancy and neonatal topics* – was developed to replace it. It may be helpful to describe such significant changes to the SMQ search strategy content and its impact on the data in the analyses and reports.

The retrieved data from applying an SMQ is not the final dataset or final answer to the query. It does not constitute the safety profile for the product without further medical review. Importantly, identification of cases with an SMQ does not confirm a causal relation between the suspect drug and the reaction(s) of interest.

III.E. Customized searches

Customizing queries when published SMQs are not suitable for an intended query

Although there are 98 SMQs (level-1 SMQs) in MedDRA v18.0, there will be situations when a published SMQ does not fully satisfy the search strategy. Instead of gathering entirely new search terms, it may be more expedient to modify an existing SMQ or combine relevant SMQs. In such situations, it is necessary to document the rationale for, and details of, changes that have been made and include such documentation when producing the safety report. The search must be renamed, stating that it is a "modified MedDRA query based on an SMQ", as it is no longer the original SMQ as published in the MedDRA terminology. This is essential, as a reviewer will otherwise assume that the unaltered SMQ has been used. If a customized search is intended to be re-used, it will have to be maintained in-house for future MedDRA versions since the MSSO and JMO do not maintain user-customized MedDRA searches. Please see *MedDRA data retrieval and presentation: points to consider*[2] for more information.

III.F. Conclusions and recommendations

SMQs are an important safety tool with wide applicability and can be used across the entire life cycle of a product. They enhance the quality, efficiency and harmonisation of search strategies and ultimately facilitate meaningful analysis and comparison of data. SMQs are routinely used by the biopharmaceutical industry, regulatory agencies and academia. To maximize the utility of SMQs, it is important to have complete and accurate ICSRs, sound and consistent medical coding practices, and adequate technological systems. It is also important to understand the criteria used to develop the SMQ to ensure that the outputs will meet the intended objective of the search. Users should also be familiar with the different design features of SMQs (e.g. algorithmic and hierarchical SMQs) and should appreciate the differences between SMQ scopes, designated as broad or narrow. In general, SMQs should be used in their standardised format. Users should be transparent and should pre-specify the SMQ(s) that will be employed to identify and analyse cases of interest. The rationale and methodology that are used to reduce "noise" should be carefully described. Another important point for communicating methodology and results is to specify the criteria used to focus on a final set of cases for detailed discussion. There are several ways in which SMQs are used today and many future potential uses are being evaluated. Chapter VI discusses some of these applications.

References:

[1]. MedDRA term selection: points to consider. ICH-endorsed guide for MedDRA users. Release 4.10, based on MedDRA Version 18.1, September 2015.
See the relevant version on www.meddra.org

2. MedDRA data retrieval and presentation: points to consider. ICH-endorsed guide for MedDRA users on data output. Release 3.8, based on MedDRA version 17.1, September 2014.
   See the relevant version on www.meddra.org
3. Introductory guide for Standardised MedDRA Queries (SMQs), Version 18.1, MSSO-DI-6226-18.1.0, September 2015.
   See the relevant version on www.meddra.org
4. Hill R, Hopstadius J, Lerch M, Noren GN. An attempt to expedite signal detection by grouping related adverse reaction terms. 24th European Medical Informatics Conference, Pisa, August 2012 (http://www.imi-protect.eu/documents/HilletalAnAttempttoExpeditSignalDetection ByGroupingRelatedAdverseReactionTerms.pdf, accessed 18 February 2016).

CHAPTER IV.
TECHNICAL ASPECTS OF IMPLEMENTATION

Executive summary

Users should have access to all the features and full functionality of SMQs for proper application – i.e. groupings of SMQ terms in hierarchical and algorithmic structures should be available to users in addition to broad and narrow term lists. This facilitates consideration of conceptually-linked terms as a group rather than being scattered in different SOCs. Tools to support use of SMQs should be largely intuitive for users. This chapter contains practical guidance on how to implement SMQs with full functionality.

IV.A. Introduction

To make proper use of SMQs in daily practice, it is of utmost importance that SMQs, including complex structures of hierarchies and algorithms, are available with full functionality for application to user databases. It is a misconception that terms in an SMQ are applied on a "copy and paste" basis to identify and retrieve the cases associated with them. The results lead to summary outputs known from the "standard" way of data presentation – i.e. in accordance with the SOC hierarchy provided in the original MedDRA structure. Groupings of SMQ terms – not only broad and narrow terms but also hierarchical and algorithmic structures – are obscured with this approach. However, a clearer view of increased frequencies may be obtained if similar terms are considered combined when compared with cases where similar terms are scattered in different SOCs. In the latter instance, there may be a perception that the terms are separate and not conceptually linked.

Data presentation in line with SMQ structures provides an additional way of keeping terms together, as described in guidance documents. Implementation of SMQ structures similar to what is already possible for the original MedDRA files would even allow spreadsheets across all SMQs, or simply an opportunity to choose the appropriate SMQ instead of copying and pasting terms separately for an SMQ each time a search is done. Routine pharmacovigilance work with SMQs may be obviated if computer tools are too challenging to users and not readily available.

IV.B. Practical guidance for implementing SMQs

The current structure of SMQ files is described in detail in the respective guidance documents. There is one major difference between SOC-Hierarchy-file (provided in file "mdhier.asc") and the SMQ hierarchical levels (provided in file "SMQ list.asc"). In the mdhier.asc file, all hierarchy levels above PT level are completely provided for all PTs line-by-line. This means that, for each PT code and name, upper levels are provided – i.e. for HLT, HLGT and SOC; other included information is ignored here because it has no relevance to the hierarchical structure. If this file is uploaded to a database, the user can create an output (e.g. for PT *Hepatic cirrhosis*, as in Table IV.B.1).

Table IV.B.1. Example for output of SOC hierarchy for a given PT *

PT CODE	PT NAME	HLT CODE	HLT NAME	HLT CODE	HLT NAME	tSOCCODE	SOC NAME
10019641	Hepatic cirrhosis	10019669	Hepatic fibrosis and cirrhosis	10019669	Hepatic fibrosis and cirrhosis	10019805	Hepato-biliary disorders

* See also changes in the current SMQ version.

All hierarchical information is thus provided in one line. Since most regulatory and company databases are designed and structured in accordance with the provisions outlined in the respective ICH documents for ICSR exchange, storage and processing, a database table is available where adverse event information is captured for each ICSR. This is done line by line for each adverse event stored for a case and is similar to the structure shown in Table IV.B.2 (only most frequently retrieved codes are stored).

Table IV.B.2. Example for output of a case safety report

Report ID	PT CODE	Other information linked to that PT, e.g. outcome
ID	10019641	Fatal

This structure allows for easy creation of structured query language (SQL) statements that attach hierarchical SOC information to each PT of a given case by simply linking PT codes of the ICSR to the identical PT code of the SOC hierarchy, resulting in a line such as illustrated in Table IV.B.3.

Table IV.B.3. Example for output of SOC hierarchy for a given PT linked to a case report *

REPORT ID	PT CODE	OUTCOME	PT NAME	HLT CODE	HLT NAME	HLT CODE	HLT NAME	SOC CODE	SOC NAME
ID	10019641	fatal	Hepatic cirrhosis	10019669	Hepatic fibrosis and cirrhosis	10019669	Hepatic fibrosis and cirrhosis	10019805	Hepatobiliary disorders

* See also changes in the current SMQ version.

A user who wishes to do the same for the SMQ hierarchy for the same PT may become confused since no file provides the SMQ structure for a given PT in the same way as the SOC hierarchy. The following description illustrates the differences.

SMQ hierarchy information is provided in two files: the SMQ list file "smq_list.asc" and the SMQ content file "smq_content.asc".

For the following examples, the only data fields provided are those that are necessary to understand how hierarchy information is provided. The SMQ list file contains important fields that are relevant for describing the SMQ hierarchy, which are the SMQ code, the SMQ name and the SMQ level. The information for different sublevel-1 SMQ names and levels is provided line by line. An example of such a hierarchy is presented in Table IV.B.4.

Table IV.B.4. Representation of hierarchical levels in the SMQ list file *

SMQ CODE	SMQ NAME	SMQ LEVEL
2000005	Hepatic disorders	1
2000006	Drug related hepatic disorders – comprehensive search	2
2000007	Drug related hepatic disorders - severe events only	3
20000013	Hepatic failure, fibrosis and cirrhosis and other liver damage-related conditions	4

* See also changes in the current SMQ version.

One pertinent question is: how can the hierarchical information be extracted from these files and brought into a structure similar to the SOC hierarchy information? To understand which hierarchical information is necessary, the charts provided in the *SMQ introductory guide* [1] should be considered. For the example of PT *Hepatic cirrhosis*, the following hierarchy should be used, as shown in Figure IV.B.1.

Figure IV.B.1. Hierarchical structure of SMQ *Hepatic disorders* (MedDRA v18.0) *

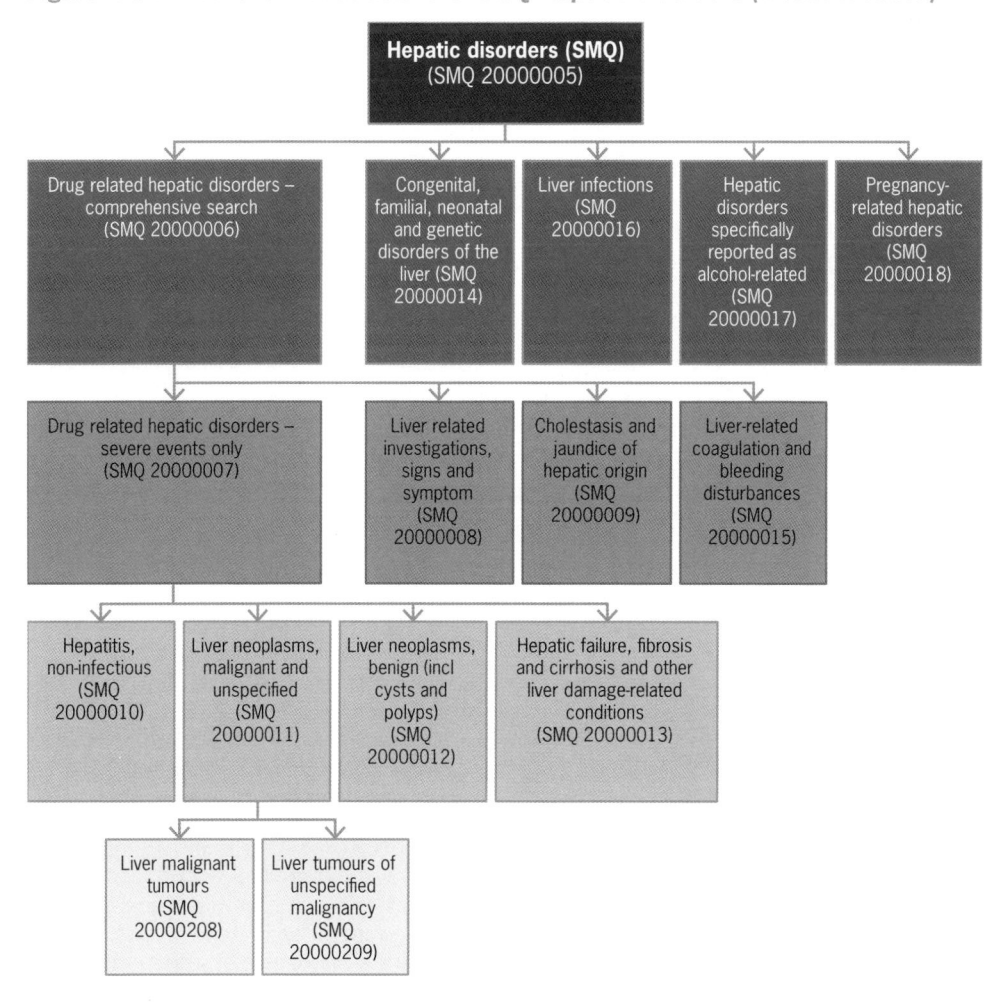

* This figure is valid for the MedDRA version given, but please see also the current MedDRA/SMQ version.

The data for the hierarchical assignment of PT *Hepatic cirrhosis* have to be taken from the SMQ content file. These data also allow for differentiation between codes which indicate an SMQ or a PT/LLT.

Table IV.B.5. Example for data output from the SMQ content file

SMQ CODE	TERM CODE	TERM LEVEL	TERM CATEGORY	TERM SCOPE
20000013	10019641	4	A	2
20000007	20000013	0	S	0
20000006	20000007	0	S	0
20000005	20000006	0	S	0

The SMQ content file contains information on PT and LLT codes which always begin with "1", while SMQ codes always begin with "2". The distinction can also be made by using field term level, which contains "4" for PTs, "5" for LLTs and 0 for SMQ codes, as well as by using field term scope (always "0" for SMQ codes, "1" for broad terms, "2" for narrow terms). In addition, the term category is indicated with "S" for SMQ codes. From these codes, no information can be derived as to which level within the hierarchy is indicated by the SMQ code. Thus, information from both files – SMQ list and SMQ content – needs to be combined to obtain the complete hierarchical information for a term extracted from the database. The steps depicted in Figure IV.B.2 are necessary.

Figure IV.B.2. Relation between SMQ list and content file to extract hierarchy information *

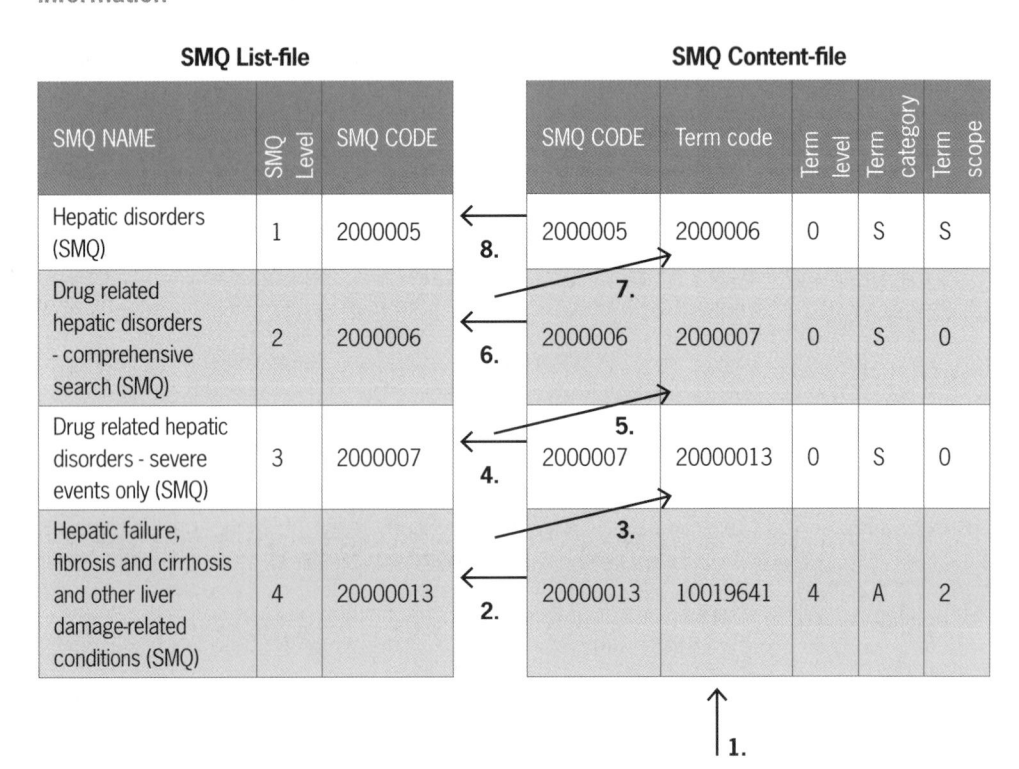

SMQ List-file				SMQ Content-file				
SMQ NAME	SMQ Level	SMQ CODE		SMQ CODE	Term code	Term level	Term category	Term scope
Hepatic disorders (SMQ)	1	2000005	8.	2000005	2000006	0	S	S
Drug related hepatic disorders - comprehensive search (SMQ)	2	2000006	6.	2000006	2000007	0	S	0
Drug related hepatic disorders - severe events only (SMQ)	3	2000007	4.	2000007	20000013	0	S	0
Hepatic failure, fibrosis and cirrhosis and other liver damage-related conditions (SMQ)	4	20000013	2.	20000013	10019641	4	A	2

↑ 1.

* This figure is valid for the MedDRA version given, but please see also the current MedDRA/SMQ version.

The numbered steps depicted in Figure IV.B.2 are further explained:

1. If there is a PT or LLT for which the hierarchical assignment is sought, the first step is to look for the PT code in the "Term code" column of the SMQ content file. Term level should be 4 or 5 (i.e. PT or LLT) respectively (in this example, PT code 10019641 with term level 4, PT/LLT *Hepatic cirrhosis*).

2. In the column labelled "SMQ CODE" on the same line, the next level up the hierarchy is indicated by the numerical value 20000013 in this example. With this SMQ code value, the SMQ list file is searched to identify the SMQ code which provides information about the SMQ level and name. If at this stage the SMQ level is indicated by "1", this would mean that there is only a one-level SMQ with assigned terms and no further hierarchical structure. If the SMQ level is greater than "1", this would mean that the code indicates a sub-SMQ further down the hierarchy. In the example, the SMQ level field is indicated by a "4" so that additional searches are necessary to obtain complete information about the hierarchy. To do so, step 3 is necessary.

3. At step 3, one goes back to the SMQ content file to look for the SMQ code in the term code field one line above. On this line, the term code, i.e. the SMQ level-4 code, corresponds to another SMQ code (20000007 in the example shown in Figure IV.B.2).

4. This code is searched for again in the SMQ list file. The corresponding line in Figure IV.B.2 indicates that the SMQ code is 20000007 and corresponds to a level-3 SMQ.

   Steps 5 and 6, as well as steps 7 and 8, respectively follow a similar strategy as already described for steps 3 and 4. At the very end, an SMQ name (or SMQ code) must be reached in the SMQ list file for each PT/LLT with entry "1" in the corresponding SMQ level field of the line found. Entry "1" in the SMQ level field means that the highest hierarchical level for a particular term has been identified (and is the only one available for non-hierarchical SMQs). Depending on the number of hierarchical levels, the number of steps needed to obtain the whole hierarchy for a given term differs – i.e. eight steps for PT/LLT that is assigned to an SMQ with four hierarchical levels (this example), 10 steps for terms of an SMQ with five hierarchical levels, six steps for a three-level hierarchy or only two steps for terms of an SMQ with no hierarchical components.

   Because of the structure of SMQ files (SMQ content and SMQ list file) it is obvious that, compared with the SOC structure, information about the hierarchical assignment of PTs/LLTs in SMQs often has to be taken from more than one line within the SMQ files to obtain the complete hierarchical information. If the steps described are taken for all SMQ terms, regardless whether a hierarchical assignment actually exists for a given term, a file can be created with one line for each term providing, if available, the hierarchical information from the SMQ list file with further information for the PT/LLT of the SMQ content file. Fields for hierarchical information that are not relevant for a PT/LLT (i.e. when the level does not exist) are left empty (which may apply to levels 2 to 5). Level-1 information is available for all terms. A possible structure is shown in Table IV.B.6. Descriptions of the SMQs and further fields from the SMQ list file may be added to this structure, as appropriate.

Table IV.B.6. Structure and source fields of a combined file of SMQ list and content file resulting in an SMQ hierarchy file

FIELD NAME	SOURCE
SMQ CODE LEVEL-1	SMQ list file
SMQ NAME LEVEL-1	SMQ list file
SMQ CODE LEVEL-2	SMQ list file
SMQ NAME LEVEL-2	SMQ list file
SMQ CODE LEVEL-3	SMQ list file
SMQ NAME LEVEL-3	SMQ list file

FIELD NAME	SOURCE
SMQ CODE LEVEL-4	SMQ list file
SMQ NAME LEVEL-4	SMQ list file
SMQ CODE LEVEL-5	SMQ list file
SMQ NAME LEVEL-5	SMQ list file
SMQ ALGORITHM	SMQ content file
TERM CODE	SMQ content file
TERM LEVEL	SMQ content file
TERM SCOPE	SMQ content file
TERM CATEGORY	SMQ content file
TERM WEIGHT	SMQ content file
TERM STATUS	SMQ content file
TERM ADDITION VERSION	SMQ content file
TERM LAST MODIFIED VERSION	SMQ content file

With this newly-generated file, the steps to be taken for linking ICSR data to the SMQ hierarchy are similar to what has been explained for attaching hierarchical SOC information. PT codes of ICSR data are linked to the identical PT code, which is named the "term code" in the newly generated SMQ hierarchy file, as provided in the original SMQ content file. The result looks like what is shown in Table IV.B.7 when all SMQ hierarchical information is included in one line for a PT in an ICSR.

Table IV.B.7. SMQ hierarchical information linked to case data *

Report ID	PT CODE	Outcome	SMQ code level-1	SMQ name level-1	SMQ code level-2	SMQ name level-2	SMQ code level-3	SMQ name level-3	SMQ code level-4	SMQ name level-4
ID 10019641		fatal	20000005	Hepatic disorders (SMQ)	20000006	Drug related hepatic disorders comprehensive search (SMQ)	20000007	Drug related hepatic disorders - severe events only (SMQ)	20000013	Hepatic failure, fibrosis and cirrhosis and other liver damage-related conditions (SMQ)

* See also changes in the current SMQ version.

Additional fields can be added as provided for PTs and LLTs in the SMQ content file shown in Table IV.B.5, with term scope, term category, term weight and term status of particular relevance. Generation of this file needs to be supported by programming and cannot be achieved manually. The strategy shown illustrates how to extract the hierarchical information from these two files in a standardised way, regardless of whether or not a hierarchical structure exists for a given SMQ and regardless of the number of levels in the SMQ. Programmers, regardless of the technology used, may support users in creating a file with all hierarchical information for a given PT or LLT in one line by following the approach described, similar to that which is already provided for the SOC hierarchy. This file may then be linked to ICSR data the same way as described above. However, it must be kept in mind that not all MedDRA terms are linked to at least one SMQ. Nevertheless, databases provide options to deal with such circumstances.

Once such a table has been created, the requirements are fulfilled for enabling the generation of outputs to PTs, reflecting the SMQ hierarchy similar to that which is known from the SOC structure. An example of this is shown in Appendix 2.

IV.C. How to deal with algorithms

Manipulation of the SMQ import files as described is not only a way to better represent the terms according to the SMQ structure, but also a much easier way to make use of the algorithms that exist for some SMQs. Table IV.B.7 illustrates how hierarchical SMQ information may be linked to case data. Other information terms such as categories (field term category in the SMQ content file) or scope (field term scope in the SMQ content file) can also be used if these terms are included in a structured database table, as shown in Table IV.B.7. An output of ICSR data with additional SMQ information for further use is shown in Table IV.C.1.

Table IV.C.1. Information about term category and scope linked to case data *

REPORT ID	PT NAME	TERM CATEGORY	TERM SCOPE
ID	Anaphylactic reaction	A	2

* See also changes in the current SMQ version.

Use of algorithms imply that cases are selected not on the basis of particular ADRs but based on PTs that are included in certain subsets of terms, as defined in the *SMQ introductory guide,* [1] which are reported together in an ICSR. Consequently, an ICSR relevant to a query using SMQs must be identified by a combination of terms rather than by using a particular term, which differs from SMQs using the broad/narrow or hierarchical approach.

In the example in Table IV.C.2, a practical subset of data has been generated to illustrate how the data may look.

In situations where technical limitations do not support automation of the algorithm, consider performing sequential searches that gradually narrow the output.

Table IV.C.2. Example for a subset of data

REPORT ID	TERM CATEGORY
ID_0001	A
ID_0001	B
ID_0001	C
ID_0002	C
ID_0002	B
ID_0003	C
ID_0003	B
ID_0004	C
ID_0004	B
ID_0009	B

REPORT ID	TERM CATEGORY
ID_0011	B
ID_2302	D
ID_2302	B
ID_2302	D
ID_2303	C
ID_2303	D

In the example presented in Table IV.C.3, all PTs of the SMQ *Anaphylactic reaction* in the database have been screened and an output has been created, which includes the case identifier (report-id) and the term category. It should be ensured that each category is assigned at the most once per case for the selected subset of data to be analysed. This can be achieved with a so-called "distinct search" for these fields in the database. Next, a spreadsheet can be created, either in the database itself (if pivot functionalities exist) or by extraction of these data from the database and further use in suitable programs such MS Excel. The pivot table may be designed with "report id" as row header and "term category" as column header. A spreadsheet using the example data of Table IV.C.2 will look similar to that shown in Table IV.C.3.

Table IV.C.3. Spreadsheet of example data, count of terms by category per case report

	A	B	C	D	E	F
1	REPORT ID	TERM CATEGORY				RELEVANCE
2		A	B	C	D	
3	ID_0001	1	1	1		relevant (A)
4	ID_0002		1	1		relevant (B and C)
5	ID_0003		1	1		relevant (B and C)
6	ID_0004		1	1		relevant (B and C)
7	ID_0009		1			
8	ID_0010	1				relevant (A)
9	ID_2302		1		1	relevant (D and (B or C)
10	ID_2303			1	1	relevant (D and (B or C)

Since a term category exists only once per case in the selection criteria as described, the number of terms belonging to categories A, B, C or D is "1" at the most. The decision of whether or not a case should be reviewed in more detail can now be based on application of the algorithm provided for algorithmic SMQs in the documentation. For SMQ *Anaphylactic reaction*, the following algorithm is used: A or (B + C) or D + (B or C). Thus, a relevant case is one with:

▶ at least one term from category A (narrow terms: e.g. PT *Anaphylactic reaction*); or

▶ at least one term from category B (respiratory signs and symptoms: e.g. PT *Asthma*) plus at least one term from category C (signs and symptoms of the skin: e.g. PT *Rash*); or

▶ at least one term from category D (e.g. PT *Blood pressure decreased*) plus either:

— at least one term from category B (respiratory signs and symptoms: e.g. PT *Asthma*) or

— at least one term from category C (signs and symptoms of the skin: e.g. PT *Rash*).

The spreadsheet is now screened for report-identifiers where the algorithm is fulfilled. The column headed "Relevance" in Table IV.C.3 indicates in which case this is true and which of the above-mentioned options leads to the desired result. The number of terms in a case that belong to the different categories is irrelevant, since the algorithm only requires at least one term for each category that contributes to fulfilment of the algorithm. Except for category-A terms, which usually contain the narrow terms of an SMQ and which are of high relevance, it is also irrelevant whether only one (or more) of the other conditions of the algorithm is fulfilled. There is also no hierarchy between the algorithmic options, again except for category-A terms because of the reasons described.

The identification of a relevant case according to the algorithm can be done manually or be supported electronically. In the example, an Excel spreadsheet has been used and a formula has been created which applies the algorithm for each case in relation to the table cells. This approach is highly recommended, particularly in high-volume outputs where manual review is resource-intensive and might easily lead to errors. In the example above, the formula supporting case identification in table cell F3 for the algorithm in SMQ *Anaphylactic reaction* could be:

=IF(B3=1;"relevant (A)"; IF(AND(C3=1;D3=1);"relevant (B and C)";IF(AND(E3=1;OR(C3=1;D3=1));"relevant (D and (B or C))";"")))

In this example, the formula has been copied to table cells F4 to F10 with enabled automated adaptation of the formula in relation to the table cells (auto complete) to initiate the check for each case. The approach described for SMQ *Anaphylactic reaction* is in principle suitable for all other algorithmic SMQs as well. However, the algorithm established may differ between SMQs so that electronic implementation of the algorithm to be applied must be handled with care.

IV.D. Algorithmic SMQs using weight factors

The SMQ *Systemic lupus erythematosus* is an algorithmic SMQ too but makes use of weight factors in addition to term categories. The approach to identifying cases with categories is very similar to other algorithms. The difference is that data field "weight-factor" is also covered by the selected data subset, as shown in Table IV.D.1.

Table IV.D.1. Example for subset of data for SMQ *Systemic lupus erythematosus*

Report ID	TERM CATEGORY	TERM WEIGHT
ID_1	H	3
ID_2	F	1
ID_2	A	0
ID_2	E	3
ID_2	H	3
ID_2	I	3
ID_3	H	3
ID_4	H	3
ID_5	H	3
ID_6	H	3
ID_7	H	3
ID_8	D	3
ID_8	A	0

Report ID	TERM CATEGORY	TERM WEIGHT
ID_9	A	0
ID_9	I	3
ID_9	E	3
ID_10	H	3
ID_11	E	3
ID_11	A	0
ID_12	E	3
ID_13	A	0
ID_14	A	0
ID_14	I	3
ID_15	A	0
ID_16	G	2
ID_17	F	1
ID_17	A	0
ID_17	I	3
ID_18	A	0
ID_19	A	0
ID_19	I	3
ID_19	F	1
ID_20	I	3
ID_20	A	0
ID_20	D	3
ID_21	H	3

The resulting spreadsheet in Table IV.D.2 resembles the one constructed for SMQ *Anaphylactic reaction*: report-id as row header, categories as column headers and the sum of weight factors for each case and category with the line total for each case. In accordance with the weight factors assigned and described in the *SMQ introductory guide*,[1] the total value needs to be "0" or greater than or equal to 7 (>=7) for a case to be considered relevant for the scope of this SMQ.

Table IV.D.2. Spreadsheet of example data, sum of weight factors by category per case report

	A	B	C	D	E	F	G	H	I	J	K	L
1	REPORT ID	TERM CATEGORY									TOTAL	RELEVANCE
2		A	B	C	D	E	F	G	H	I		
3	ID_1								3		3	
4	ID_2	0				3	1		3	3	10	relevant (A)
5	ID_3								3		3	
6	ID_4								3		3	
7	ID_5								3		3	
8	ID_6								3		3	
9	ID_7								3		3	
10	ID_8	0			3						3	relevant (A)
11	ID_9	0				3				3	6	relevant (A)
12	ID_10								3		3	
13	ID_11	0			3						3	relevant (A)
14	ID_12				3						3	
15	ID_13	0									0	relevant (A)
16	ID_14	0								3	3	relevant (A)
17	ID_15	0									0	relevant (A)
18	ID_16							2			2	
19	ID_17	0					1			3	4	relevant (A)
20	ID_18	0									0	relevant (A)
21	ID_19	0					1			3	4	relevant (A)
22	ID_20	0			3					3	6	relevant (A)
23	ID_21								3		3	

Review of the spreadsheet can again be done manually or can be supported by electronic means, as explained above. The formula applied here in the Excel sheet for column L3 reads as follows:

=IF(AND(B3=0;ISNUMBER(B3));"relevant (A)";IF(SUM (C3:H3)>=7;"relevant (sum weight-factors >=7)";""))

and must be copied to all lines with report numbers – i.e. to columns L4 to L23 with adaptation to the table cells for each case (auto complete).

In this example, only cases with terms from category A (i.e. narrow terms) were retrieved as relevant for further review.

IV.E. Conclusions and recommendations

The current SMQ structure and tools provide improved selection of relevant terms and their application in search strategies. Application of algorithms and data presentation according to the SMQ structure is not supported in the same way. The approach shown provides additional possibilities for data analysis, retrieval and presentation since the SMQ structure is attached in a similar way to that which is currently possible with the SOC structure. Application of existing algorithms and implementation of new ones, if being developed, becomes easier.

References:

1. Introductory guide for Standardised MedDRA Queries (SMQs), Version 18.1, MSSO-DI-6226-18.1.0, September 2015. See the relevant version on www.meddra.org

CHAPTER V.
COMMUNICATION OF RESULTS

Executive summary

This chapter describes points to consider when preparing a report of output from the application of an SMQ to a safety database. It also includes recommendations for analysis of the search results and production of a complete answer to the query posed. The final documentation should enable the search to be reproduced if necessary. Table A.3.1 in Appendix 3 shows a list of items to be considered when communicating the results of a query.

V.A. General considerations for communication of search results

It is important to convey the question being addressed, the methodology used, results obtained, and interpretation of the output of the query in a logical and concise manner. The following sections might be considered for a report, although this approach can be modified according to the specific situation.

V.B. Points to consider when preparing a report with query output

This section outlines proposed content to consider when preparing a report to communicate the results of a query. A template that corresponds to the points below is presented in Appendix 3. Parenthetic numbering that appears in this section refers to sections of the report template, but numbering and content may be modified to fit the circumstances of the report.

- ### V.B.i. Executive summary

This unnumbered section of the report should include a very brief summary of the question, its origin, and an overview of the search strategy, results and overall conclusion.

- ### V.B.ii. Background for the question being addressed (Template section 1.)

Introduction (Template section 1.a.)
This section may describe the following points: the specific request, the source of the request, historical aspects and time window relevant to the request, and the objective of the report. In addition, it would be appropriate to include commentary on the relevance of the request to any related conditions that appear in the reference safety information (e.g. regulator-approved prescribing information).

Medicinal product (or medical device, etc. as appropriate) (Template section 1.b.)

This section may provide summary information – such as indication, formulation, posology, mechanism of action – on medicinal product(s), whether still in clinical development or already marketed. The information may come from the Investigator Brochure or product label information (summary of product characteristics, prescribing information, product monograph, or package insert). If this involves a comparison of more than one medical product, the basis for selection of the comparator products should be briefly stated along with their characteristics, as above. Consideration should be given to including estimates of population exposure (divided according to clinical trials and post-marketing, as appropriate) to provide context for the number of cases retrieved by the query.

Medical condition of interest (Template section 1.c.)

A clear definition of the medical condition being evaluated should be provided in this section, which includes a brief description of the natural history of the condition, profiling the manifestations over time, signs, symptoms and usual treatments (since they may serve as confounders in the search). The description should indicate the breadth of the condition which may (or may not) include very nonspecific signs or symptoms such as abdominal pain, aching joints, etc. When appropriate, references from the scientific literature can be included. All aspects of the medical condition should be described in the context of SMQ documentation – i.e. how the definition provided in the *Introductory guide for standardised MedDRA queries* [1] applies to the medical condition of interest.

• V.B.iii. Methods (Template section 2.)

Search and selection strategy (Template section 2.a.)

This section should include a precise description of the intended scope of the query.

MedDRA version of the SMQ (Template section 2.b.)

Since it is essential to match the MedDRA version of the SMQ to the MedDRA version of the MedDRA-coded database, the version should be specified in both instances. Similarly, if applying a modified SMQ or in-house/ad hoc query, the search terms should be from the same MedDRA version as the data, and the version number should be specified in the report. Ideally, if the data are in a MedDRA version that predates the production release of the SMQ being applied, one may wish to consider recoding the data in a later MedDRA version before conducting the search. Whether recoding is appropriate may depend on the reason for the query.

SMQ utilized (Template section 2.c.)

If an SMQ is used, the name of the level-1/parent SMQ or sub-SMQs for hierarchical SMQs should be provided. The scope applied (narrow, broad) should also be specified. For algorithmic SMQs and the SMQ with term weightings, one should state whether the algorithm or weightings were applied. If more than one SMQ was used, this should be stated.

SMQ modified (or in-house/ad hoc query) (Template section 2.d.)

If an SMQ has been modified because it did not meet the requirements of the query, modifications should be described in the report. The modified SMQ should not be described as an SMQ but as a modified query based on an SMQ. If the modified query is re-applied in the future, the query will have to be up-versioned by the user to match the MedDRA version of the data being searched.

Data sources (Template section 2.e.)

The ICSRs being evaluated should be categorized (e.g. ICSRs from organized data collection schemes, clinical trials, observational studies, spontaneous reports [including geographical origins], serious/non-serious, medically confirmed or not, and whether causality was assessed). Further, it would be important to know if there are limitations on the number of PTs allowed in coding.

When multiple sources of data are queried (e.g. co-development, licensing arrangements, mergers, etc.), different MedDRA coding conventions may have been used over time and it would be appropriate to assess the potential for confounders in this section, as well as relevant information on data migration and MedDRA versioning practices.

If MedDRA-coded data have been extracted from other sources, this should be described, as should the coding conventions and other relevant information such as legacy data migration or conversions over time. If epidemiology (observational data) is included, there may be a need for mapping between the terminology (e.g. ICD-9) utilized by the epidemiology databases (e.g. health-care records) and MedDRA.

Medical assessment (Template section 2.f.)

The process for medical assessment of query output should be described, including any steps to enhance review on cases of interest (i.e. validation or triage). Likewise, efforts to reduce "noise" in the data available for medical review should be described, as should the justification.

• V.B.iv. Results of query (Template section 3.)

Overview (Template section 3.a.)

Provide a high-level summary of the number of cases retrieved, the time window, the type of data (clinical, spontaneous, whether medically confirmed, etc.).

Case presentation (Template section 3.b.)

This section should include individual summaries of relevant cases. If appropriate and relevant, cases that are not considered to be contributory to addressing the query may also be summarized before being excluded from further discussion. The criteria used for excluding any cases retrieved with the SMQ should be provided.

In all cases, the limitations of the data should be clearly described. These include the likely occurrence of missing data and the effects of different coding practices (i.e. diagnosis/syndrome vs. sign or symptom).

Summary of data (Template section 3.c.)

This section can be used to consolidate query findings.

Additional relevant information (Template section 3.d.)

Include known or suspected information, such as potential confounders that may influence the interpretation of query results as presented in the report.

• V.B.v. Discussion and conclusion of report (Template section 4.)

Provide discussion of results of data searches and their interpretation with a conclusion. In most situations, the findings resulting from use of SMQs will provide a series of cases that are retrieved on the basis of the presence of one or more PTs in the coded case. As a rule, the information supports hypothesis generation, rather than hypothesis strengthening or proof. Nevertheless, the occurrence of the cluster of PTs in an SMQ, along with the demographics of the cases, can be useful in the design of structured clinical and/or epidemiological studies to test these hypotheses, and this should be noted in suggesting future studies.

- **V.B.vi. References (Template section 5.)**

When relevant, provide references from the scientific literature. References may be particularly useful in describing the medical condition of interest and in supporting modifications to the published SMQ.

V.C. Conclusions and recommendations

Presentation of results of an SMQ search in a relatively standardised format will enhance the broader adoption of SMQs in evaluation of the safety of medical products. Appendix 3 contains a list of items to be considered when communicating the results of a query. This chapter has outlined the basic steps that ideally should be considered in communicating the results of an analysis. This serves not only to provide validation of the SMQ for its purpose, but also to provide detailed guidance for future users.

References:

1. Introductory guide for Standardised MedDRA Queries (SMQs), Version 18.1, MSSO-DI-6226-18.1.0, September 2015. See the relevant version on www.meddra.org

CHAPTER VI.

CURRENT CONSIDERATIONS AND FUTURE DIRECTIONS

Executive summary

This report describes the purpose and recommended use of SMQs in medical product safety surveillance across the entire product life cycle. Examples, such as monitoring of potential safety risks and analysis of aggregate data, are included in this report. These examples are meant to illustrate the use of queries in systematic analyses (e.g. meta-analysis), interventional clinical trials, signal detection, signal assessment and other database searches. In clinical trials SMQs can be used to compare test medical products to comparators, including placebo, and to other molecules in the same pharmacologic-therapeutic class or with a similar mechanism of action. SMQs can also serve as useful tools in vaccine vigilance and technovigilance for medical devices.

In the future, there may be opportunities to apply SMQs to active safety surveillance and non-interventional studies as, for example, the use of SMQ concepts in grouping ICD and other codes (e.g. READ).

VI.A. Current considerations

In this updated publication, the CIOMS SMQ WG reports on the purpose and appropriate use of SMQs in medical product safety surveillance activities. It is hoped that the activities of different stakeholders involved in biopharmaceutical and other medical product development and surveillance will benefit from the use of SMQs. This report enhances key information from the original edition and also shares the experience gained in the development and applications of SMQs since the publication of that report.

SMQs have several benefits to MedDRA subscribers, including:

- a standardised communication that facilitates comparison of safety data across products and between organizations;
- consistency of data retrieval strategy over time; and
- continuous maintenance and update of SMQs with each new MedDRA version.

SMQs have three basic design features, namely:

- narrow/broad;
- algorithmic; and
- hierarchical.

These are not mutually exclusive. The term content for almost all SMQs consists of both narrow scope terms and broad scope terms and may incorporate additional design features.

The narrow-scope terms bestow specificity and the broad-scope terms sensitivity to the search results. The idea behind an algorithmic SMQ is that a case is more likely to be of interest if it contains a defined combination of broad terms than if it contains a single broad term. Hierarchical SMQs relate to one another in a hierarchical relationship. The hierarchy consists of one or more subordinate SMQs that are combined to create a superordinate, more inclusive SMQ.

▶ In Chapter IV a more detailed technical description of the three different basic types of SMQs is presented including practical examples. Examples of SMQ development are also presented in Appendix 2. These examples were selected to illustrate various aspects of SMQ development and are intended to provide practical and detailed aspects of SMQ development. All developed SMQs were tested against products for which the medical condition of interest was mentioned in the product labelling or emerged during post-marketing.

- ## VI.A.i. Consensus on harmonised approaches

The CIOMS WGs included very specialized expertise and major achievements have been reached. At the time of the introduction of MedDRA v18.0, there were 98 SMQ topics (level-1 SMQs) available that contain another 116 sub-SMQs within them (hierarchical SMQs), see Sections I.A, II.H and II.K.

Application of an SMQ search strategy is recommended as a first step in an assessment phase; completion of the task of retrieval of cases of interest using an SMQ involves review of the retrieved data. Stakeholders planning to use SMQs are advised to consider the bullet points below. In addition, users should check that the data to be searched are all coded with the same version of MedDRA and that the SMQ version is identical to the MedDRA version used for coding the data.

When SMQs are used as tools, the following should be considered:

▶ Review the list of available SMQs through a browser and select one or more that applies to the question being posed.

▶ Use the *SMQ introductory guide*[1] (see Chapter II) to obtain information – e.g. definition (the definition of the concept that the SMQ was designed to address is particularly important), intent, expected query results – about the selected SMQ(s).

▶ Review the term content of an SMQ (term content consists of PTs) to ensure that these are relevant to the medical issue/condition.

- ## VI.A.ii. Stakeholders

Safety surveillance is practised by regulatory authorities, academic/scientific institutions, pharmaceutical companies and others involved in biopharmaceutical and medical product development and use.

VI.B. Future directions

SMQs can be applied throughout the life cycle of a product to provide a meaningful safety profile. Examples of settings in which SMQs can be applied to data coded in MedDRA have been addressed in Chapters II and III. These include monitoring of potential safety risks and analysis of aggregate data, including systematic analyses (e.g. meta-analysis) in interventional clinical trials and signal detection, and case searches and alerts, including periodic reporting of aggregate data in post-marketing safety assessments. In clinical trials SMQs can be used to compare medical products with comparators, including placebo, and with other molecules in the same pharmacologic-therapeutic class or with a similar mechanism of action.

SMQs can also serve as tools in vaccine vigilance and in technovigilance for medical devices.

Although new SMQs have been requested by MedDRA subscribers through a change request process administered by the MSSO and JMO in association with an ICH Advisory Panel, other mechanisms may become available in the future. Subscribers are encouraged to submit future change requests for existing

SMQs and for creation of new SMQs (including those queries developed within a subscriber organization that may be useful to others).

The results of SMQ searches are primarily useful to clarify hypotheses and provide guidance to more structured epidemiological studies or clinical trials by helping to define endpoints and, in some cases, populations at risk and confounders. In the future, there may be more opportunities to apply the SMQ approach to active safety surveillance and non-interventional studies and apply this to groupings of ICD codes and data coded with other terminologies. Epidemiologists, pharmacoepidemiologists and pharmacoeconomists utilize ICD codes to characterize a disorder. SMQs often provide a broader clinical description than is available in non-MedDRA-coded datasets. In the future, it could be useful to apply the concepts embodied within SMQs to such data after mapping the relevant non-MedDRA terms to MedDRA. Such use might facilitate the analysis of large pools of data from disparate sources for safety or other purposes.

Considerations for the future include:

- impact(s) of future SMQ enhancements on all aspects of safety surveillance science;
- requirements for future SMQ work, including maintenance and the evolution of MedDRA;
- strategies to drive optimal use of SMQs to better protect patient safety and public health; and
- opportunities and challenges in considering global appetite and capacity for SMQ application.

References:

1. Introductory guide for Standardised MedDRA Queries (SMQs), Version 18.1, MSSO-DI-6226-18.1.0, September 2015. See the relevant version on www.meddra.org

APPENDICES

APPENDIX 1. MEMBERSHIP AND WORKING PROCEDURES OF THE CIOMS SMQ WORKING GROUPS

APPENDIX 2. EXAMPLES OF SMQ DEVELOPMENT
2.a. SMQ *Rhabdomyolysis/myopathy*
2.b. SMQ *Anaphylactic reaction*
2.c. SMQ *Hepatic disorders*

APPENDIX 3. COMMUNICATION OF SEARCH RESULTS

APPENDIX 1.

MEMBERSHIP AND WORKING PROCEDURES OF THE CIOMS SMQ WORKING GROUPS

SMQs have been developed as a result of a partnership between ICH, CIOMS and other stakeholders after a need was identified for strategies and tools for retrieval of MedDRA-coded clinical safety data. This CIOMS activity has been conducted in conjunction with the ICH MMB. SMQs represent a standardised approach to establishing a baseline for the identification of ICSRs that may represent defined medical conditions with the potential to impact benefit–risk evaluations. Following an organizational meeting in May 2002, a CIOMS Working Group on the Rational Use of MedDRA Terminology for Drug Safety Database Searches was established in September of that year. The original 24 members were senior scientists representing seven regulatory authorities, seven pharmaceutical companies and other organizations (e.g. WHO and CIOMS). Subsequently, the MedDRA MSSO and the JMO joined the group and a decision was taken to consolidate efforts, such that work on SMQs would subsume development of other cooperative data query efforts – i.e. work on SSCs and MAGs would be phased out. The joint collaborative effort was designed to take full advantage of technical expertise, administrative functions, access to MedDRA-coded regulatory and company databases, distribution services, and maintenance capabilities. In May 2003 the reconstituted Working Group was renamed the CIOMS Working Group on SMQs.

In November 2004, the workplan of the CIOMS WG was revised to adopt a regular cadence of SMQ production.

The WG designed and adopted a process to facilitate a consistent and uniform approach to SMQ development, documentation and subsequent testing by the WG (and field testing by stakeholders). The initial process adopted by the WG is described in Chapter II of the CIOMS WG report *SMQs development and rational use of standardised MedDRA queries (SMQs).*[1] The ICH MMB endorsed this multistep, iterative development and testing process for SMQs. Subsequently, an SMQ IWG was formed to continue development and testing of additional SMQs and to produce a second edition of that report (known as the *SMQ "Red book"*)[1] that builds on experience with SMQ use and practical aspects of SMQ implementation.

Historical milestones are summarized in Table A.1.1.

Table A.1.1. Milestones for SMQ development by the CIOMS Working Group, as of November 2004 (with subsequent modification)[A]

Milestones	Date	Target number of new named SMQs	
		Total proposed or planned	Cumulative number to be completed
CIOMS Working Group inception	Sep 2002	97	-
Initial SMQs finalized	May 2005	59	15
Second batch SMQs finalized	May 2006	60	30
Additional milestones	May 2007	60	45
Additional milestones	May 2008	60	60
Additional milestones	May 2009	60	74
Additional milestones	May 2010	60	82
Additional milestones	May 2011	60	90[B]

[A] Target numbers of SMQs in Table A.1.1 do not necessarily represent numbers of distinct queries that the WG Core Group eventually included in a scientifically-sound SMQ package – in other words, concepts for named SMQ packages are displayed on subsequent tables, but the WG Core Group found it logical to produce a single named SMQ package (i.e. level-1 SMQs) with distinct subqueries (i.e. SMQs at levels 2 to 5). This approach subsumes certain medical concepts while at the same time allowing for incorporation of subscriber requests and assimilation of concepts in MedDRA's former SSCs. Table A.1.1 has not been updated since May 2011.
[B] Note that 94 level-1 SMQs were published with MedDRA v16.1 as of October 2013.

The relevant CIOMS development teams established work teams and timelines for each SMQ and these groups accomplished the associated tasks through ad hoc email exchanges, scheduled teleconferences and regular face-to-face meetings. The composition of the WG, the WG Core Group and the IWG is listed in Table A.1.2; each group comprised senior scientists from the listed organizations. The schedule of face-to-face meetings of the CIOMS WGs is shown in Table A.1.3.

Table A.1.2. Members, advisors and observers who have contributed to the development of SMQs as part of the CIOMS SMQ Working Groups (2002–2016)[A]

Name	Organizational affiliation at first participation
Walter Aellig	Novartis Pharma AG
Silvia Bader-Weder	F. Hoffman-La Roche
Cecilia Birell	Uppsala Monitoring Center
Michael Blum	Wyeth
Mariette Boerstoel	Organon
Thomas Bold	Merck
Sonja Brajovic	Food and Drug Administration (USA)
Miles Braun	Food and Drug Administration (USA)
Gunilla Brenning	Medical Products Agency (Sweden)
Elliot Brown	Elliot Brown Consulting Ltd.

APPENDIX 1. MEMBERSHIP AND WORKING PROCEDURES OF THE CIOMS SMQ WORKING GROUPS

Name	Organizational affiliation at first participation
Anne Castot	Agence française de sécurité sanitaire des produits de santé (France)
Mary Couper	World Health Organization
Isolde Crusius	Boehringer-Ingelheim
Jingying-Jean Cui	Wyeth
Morell David	Medicines Control Agency (United Kingdom)
Vikram Dev	AstraZeneca
David Dressler	Merck
Agostino Faggiotto	Pharmacia
Paul Fallot	Schering-Plough
Ann Gaines	Food and Drug Administration (USA)
Stuart Geary	Eisai
Shelley Ghandi	Medicines and Healthcare products Regulatory Agency (United Kingdom)
William Gregory	Pfizer
Gregory Gribko	Pfizer
Ilona Grosse-Michaelis	Bayer-Schering AG/Bayer Pharmaceuticals AG
Isabelle Gueller	International Council for Harmonisation, Secretariat
Osamu Handa	Japanese Maintenance Organization/Society of Japanese Pharmacopoeia
David Henley	Eli Lilly
Astrid Herpers	F. Hoffman-La Roche
Wakako Horiki	Pharmaceuticals and Medical Devices Agency (Japan)
Juhana Idänpään-Heikkilä†	Council for International Organizations of Medical Sciences
Sonoko Ishihara	Pharmaceuticals and Medical Devices Agency (Japan)
Kerstin Jansson	Medical Products Agency (Sweden)
Judith Jones	The Degge Group Ltd.
Anne Kehely	Lilly UK
Brigitte Keller-Stanislawski	Paul Ehrlich Institute
Jean Kilgour-Christie	Eli Lilly
Tatsuo Kishi	Pharmaceuticals and Medical Devices Agency (Japan)
Chie Kojima	Ministry of Health, Labour and Welfare (Japan)
Jürgen Köster	Boehringer-Ingelheim
Gerhard Kremer	Boehringer-Ingelheim
Gottfried Kreutz	Federal Institute for Drugs and Medical Devices (Germany), Council for International Organizations of Medical Sciences
Katja Kusche	F. Hoffman-La Roche
Gary Lacey	Therapeutic Goods Administration (Australia)
Magnus Lerch	Schering AG

APPENDIX 1. MEMBERSHIP AND WORKING PROCEDURES OF THE CIOMS SMQ WORKING GROUPS

Name	Organizational affiliation at first participation
Jin Ling	Eli Lilly
Susan Lu	Food and Drug Administration (USA)
Sabine Luik	Boehringer-Ingelheim
Lynn Macdonald	Health Canada
Kerri MacKay	Therapeutic Goods Administration (Australia)
Harumi Maniwa	Pharmaceuticals and Medical Devices Agency (Japan)
Kazuhiro Matsui	Ministry of Health Labor and Welfare (Japan)
Arthur Meiners	Johnson & Johnson
Roberta Michaelis	Wyeth
Christiane Michel	Novartis Pharma AG
Constantin Mirea	Boehringer-Ingelheim
Tomás Moreleda	MedDRA Maintenance and Support Services Organization
Odette Morin	International Council for Harmonisation, Secretariat
Jean Morrone	UCB Pharma
Patricia Mozzicato	MedDRA Maintenance and Support Services Organization
James Mundell	MedDRA Maintenance and Support Services Organization
Yutaka Nagao	Japanese Maintenance Organization/Society of Japanese Pharmacopoeia
Jugo Nermin	Pharmacia
Victoria Newbould	European Medicines Agency
Savian Nicholas	Bristol-Myers Squibb
Miki Ohta	Pharmaceuticals and Medical Devices Agency (Japan)
Norbert Paeschke	Federal Institute for Drugs and Medical Devices (Germany)
Erick Pelfrene	European Agency for the Evaluation of Medicinal Products
Christine Peric	Aventis
Lembit Rägo	Council for International Organizations of Medical Sciences
John Reed	Amgen
Christina Reith	F. Hoffman-La Roche
Patrick Revelle	MedDRA Maintenance and Support Services Organization
Bruce Robinson	Merck
Dawn Ronan	International Council for Harmonisation, Secretariat
Alex Ruggieri	Amgen
Eva-Beate Rump	MedDRA Maintenance and Support Services Organization
Yasuo Sakurai	Japanese Maintenance Organization/Society of Japanese Pharmacopoeia
Aniello Santoro	European Medicines Agency
Makan Sarkeshik	Amgen

Name	Organizational affiliation at first participation
Marina Sharayeva	Pharma-Center (Ukraine)
Kazuyuki Sekiguchi	Japanese Maintenance Organization
Gunilla Sjölin-Forsberg	Council for International Organizations of Medical Sciences
Eiko Tada	Pharmaceuticals and Medical Devices Agency (Japan)
Nogusa Takahara	Pharmaceuticals and Medical Devices Agency (Japan)
Hitomi Takeshita	Chugai Pharmaceutical Co., Ltd
Yo Tanaka	Chugai Pharmaceutical Co., Ltd
Philippe Thouvay	F. Hoffman-La Roche
Melissa Truffa	Food and Drug Administration (USA)
Panos Tsintis	European Agency for the Evaluation of Medicinal Products
Sarah Vaughan	Medicines and Healthcare products Regulatory Agency (United Kingdom)
Joachim Veith	Amgen
Jan Venulet	Council for International Organizations of Medical Sciences
Yu Wada	Pharmaceuticals and Medical Devices Agency (Japan)
Wayne Wallis	Amgen
Bill Wilson	Health Canada
Christina Winter	GlaxoSmithKline
Martina Wollenhaupt	F. Hoffman-La Roche
Hideto Yoki	National Institute of Health Sciences (Japan)
Masahiko Yokota	Pharmaceuticals and Medical Devices Agency (Japan)
Susan Yu	Amgen
Tiziana Zaccheo	Pharmacia
Anna Zhao-Wong	MedDRA Maintenance and Support Services Organization

[A] This is a cumulative list of senior scientists who have been important contributors to SMQ development over time, organized alphabetically by last name, and their associated organizations. These contributors have served as members, advisors or observers of the CIOMS SMQ Working Groups for differing periods of time; some have contributed for the full duration (2002 to 2015), while others have addressed discrete topics. In some cases organizations changed names over the course of this project or contributors changed affiliations; this is not reflected in the listing. The list generally includes the affiliation of the contributor when he or she first joined the Working Group. It is recognized that the list may inadvertently be incomplete and the editorial team apologizes, in advance, for any unintentional oversight that may have occurred.

Table A.1.3. Face-to-face meetings of the CIOMS SMQ Working Group, CIOMS SMQ Core Group, and CIOMS SMQ Implementation Working Group, as of September 2015

Meeting Number	Date	Location	Venue
0	May 2002	Frankfurt	Frankfurt Airport Sheraton
1	Sep 2002	Basle	Roche
2	Jan 2003	London	EMEA
3	May 2003	Bonn	BfArM
4	Oct 2003	London	MHRA
5	Feb 2004	Geneva	ICH/IFPMA/WHO
6	May 2004	Uppsala	MPA
7	Sep 2004	Paris	Aventis
8	Jan 2005	Washington, DC	Degge
9	May 2005	Berlin	Schering AG
10	Aug 2005	London	GlaxoSmithKline
11	Nov 2005	Geneva	ICH/IFPMA/CIOMS
12	Feb 2006	Ingelheim	Boehringer-Ingelheim
13	May 2006	Milan	Pfizer
14	Aug 2006	London	EMEA
15	Nov 2006	London	Amgen
16	Feb 2007	Arlington	Degge
17	May 2007	Geneva	ICH/IFPMA/CIOMS
18	Aug 2007	Quebec City	Health Canada
19	Nov 2007	Basle	Roche
20	Feb 2008	Basle	Novartis
21	May 2008	Geneva	ICH/IFPMA/CIOMS
Since creation of CIOMS Core Group			
22	Sep 2008	New York City	Pfizer
23	Mar 2009	Ingelheim	Boehringer-Ingelheim
24	Sep 2009	London	GlaxoSmithKline
25	Mar 2010	Bonn	BfArM
26	Sep 2010	Berlin	Bayer Schering AG
27	Mar 2011	Geneva	WHO (ICH/IFPMA/CIOMS)
Since creation of CIOMS Implementation Working Group			
28	Sep 2011	Thousand Oaks	Amgen
29	Mar 2012	Windelsham	Lilly
30	Sep 2012	London	GlaxoSmithKline
31	Apr 2013	Geneva	WHO (ICH/IFPMA/CIOMS)

Meeting Number	Date	Location	Venue
32	Oct 2013	Basel	Novartis
33	Apr 2014	Geneva	ICH/IFPMA
34	Oct 2014	Geneva	ICH/IFPMA
35	May 2015	Geneva	CIOMS
36	Sep 2015	Geneva	ICH/IFPMA
37	Mar 2016	Geneva	CIOMS

References:

1. SMQs development and rational use of Standardised MedDRA Queries (SMQs). Retrieving adverse drug reactions with MedDRA. Report of the CIOMS Working Group. Geneva: CIOMS; 2004.

APPENDIX 2.

EXAMPLES OF SMQ DEVELOPMENT

Preface

The text in the examples that follow in this appendix was taken from the original documentation prepared by the SMQ development teams testing the SMQs prior to release. Thus the terminology used within Appendix 2 may differ from that in the main body of this publication. The documentation for the SMQs reflects the observations and opinions of the SMQ development team. These examples have been selected to illustrate various aspects of SMQ development and are intended to provide practical and detailed aspects of SMQ development. Readers are reminded to use the relevant SMQ version and active SMQ terms.

- SMQ *Rhabdomyolysis/myopathy* illustrates a simple search, with concepts that are organized into a narrow search and a broad search.
- SMQ *Anaphylactic reaction* illustrates a complex algorithmic search that contains linked concepts in several different categories.
- SMQ *Hepatic disorders* illustrates a complex, hierarchical search that includes several grouped subsearches.

These examples provide a snapshot in time and should not be construed as representing the current state of the named level-1 SMQ. As noted in Chapters I and II, the MSSO publishes two versions of MedDRA each year to reflect updates and agreed changes in the terminology. SMQs are maintained in alignment with each MedDRA version. Changes in the terminology that have an impact on SMQs are documented in a Version Report for each MedDRA release. One section of the Version Report focuses on the changes that apply at the SMQ level (e.g. new SMQs, renamed SMQs, etc.) and another section reflects changes in SMQs at the PT level. The Version Report compares changes from the current and previous MedDRA versions.

For a comprehensive set of SMQ changes, an online MVAT which compares any two MedDRA versions, including nonconsecutive versions, provides the same reports. This tool is available to all MedDRA subscribers.

As indicated in Chapter II, SMQ users are reminded to select an appropriate SMQ, carefully review the documentation provided for the SMQ of interest and match the version of the SMQ to the MedDRA version used to code the target data.

APPENDIX 2.a. Example of SMQ development: SMQ *Rhabdomyolysis/myopathy*

• A.2.a.A. Background on rhabdomyolysis and myopathy

Myopathy is a disorder of striated muscle, with or without changes in muscle mass, and may be accompanied by muscle pain or tenderness. [1, 2] Rhabdomyolysis is a syndrome resulting from extensive necrosis of skeletal muscle with release of muscle contents – particularly creatine kinase (CK) and other muscle enzymes (such as aminotransferases and lactic dehydrogenase), creatinine, potassium, uric acid, myoglobin, calcium and phosphorus – into the systemic circulation. [3, 4] Some cases are related to hereditary metabolic or structural abnormalities effecting skeletal muscle cells, such as disorders of glycogen and lipid metabolism. [3] However, the majority of cases occur in healthy individuals due to a variety of non-hereditary causes such as trauma (due to crushing injuries or excessive exercise), bacterial and/or viral infections (such as staphylococcus or influenza), medications (such as HMG-CoA reductase inhibitors and antipsychotics), recreational drugs (such as cocaine, amphetamines and alcohol), toxins (such as tetanus and some snake venoms) and ischemia. [3, 5]

Rhabdomyolysis varies from mild and self-limiting to severe and possibly life-threatening. [3, 4, 5] Muscle signs and symptoms usually include muscle pain, weakness, tenderness and contractures, usually involving large muscles such as those of the calves, thighs and lower back, but can also involve the chest, abdomen, palate and throat, and masticatory muscles. Other nonspecific symptoms can include weight gain, fatigue, malaise, fever, nausea, tachycardia and dark red or cola-coloured urine. Potentially serious systemic sequelae include acute renal failure, compartment syndrome, disseminated intravascular coagulation, cardiomyopathy and respiratory failure. [3, 4]

Laboratory abnormalities usually indicative of rhabdomyolysis include elevated CK, particularly the isoform originating from skeletal muscle (CK-MM, often markedly elevated), myoglobinuria and increased serum myoglobin. Other laboratory findings may include elevated serum creatinine, lactic dehydrogenase and aminotransferases. Hypocalcaemia and potentially life-threatening hyperkalemia (in patients with acute renal failure) may also occur. Diagnosis can be confirmed by muscle biopsy. [3, 4, 5]

• A.2.a.B. Methodology

MedDRA terms (MedDRA v5.1) were initially identified by a "bottom-up" search of LLTs. To make this search reasonably specific, the types of PTs identified included rhabdomyolysis or myopathy and manifestations strongly suggestive of myopathy such as myoglobinaemia or myoglobinuria. After the relevant MedDRA PTs and their place in the MedDRA hierarchy were identified, a "top-down" review was performed to identify other related and potentially relevant PTs, as well as their primary SOC allocations.

Because of the variety of clinical manifestations associated with rhabdomyolysis or myopathy, it is possible that cases may not have been initially classified and coded as such. In an attempt to provide sufficient sensitivity to this SMQ, specific events and constellations were included – such as compartment syndrome and other, non-myopathy-related muscle events (myalgia, muscle fatigue or weakness, musculoskeletal pain or discomfort, or abnormal muscle biopsy) or other non-musculoskeletal events suggestive of possible rhabdomyolysis or myopathy (renal failure and related events, increased CK or other muscle enzymes, hypocalcaemia or chromaturia). These terms were also identified with a similar "bottom-up" search followed by a "top-down" search of the terminology.

In an effort to determine how well the candidate SMQ would identify potential cases of rhabdomyolysis or myopathy, a large pharmaceutical company safety database was searched using the candidate SMQ. This company's safety database contains cases of adverse events reported spontaneously, cases reported from health authorities, cases published in the medical literature, and cases of serious adverse events reported from clinical studies and company-sponsored marketing programmes (solicited cases), regardless of causality. The database was reviewed for nonclinical study origin cases reported by healthcare professionals to the database for two of the company's products. Rhabdomyolysis was added to the labelling for the first product (Compound 1) after it had been commercially available for about two years. The database was reviewed for cases with events coded to any of the PTs listed in the candidate SMQ throughout the month that the labelling was amended to include rhabdomyolysis.

For the second product (Compound 2), rhabdomyolysis was added to the product labelling several years prior to the testing of this SMQ. The database was reviewed for cases involving Compound 2 cases with events coded to any of the PTs listed in the proposed SMQ up to the cut-off date that was used for a company review of possible drug interaction-related cases of rhabdomyolysis. For these two products, it was expected that the candidate SMQ would identify a reasonable pool of potential cases to be included in a case review.

• A.2.a.C. Results

As a result of this review (MedDRA v5.1), a total of 49 relevant PTs were identified for inclusion in the SMQ. The primary allocations for these 49 PTs have listed them under six SOCs, 12 HLGTs and 17 HLTs.

Based on the PTs identified, queries of the database to identify relevant cases for review were conducted in a two-step manner. The first step was to conduct a "narrow" search to identify a core set of cases specifically reported to involve rhabdomyolysis, myopathy or myopathy-related manifestations of muscle necrosis, myoglobinaemia or myoglobinuria. This first search involved the nine rhabdomyolysis- or myopathy-related PTs listed in Table A.2.a.1. In an effort to make the query relatively specific, not all possibly rhabdomyolysis- or myopathy-related events were included (for instance, not all PTs listed under the HLT *Myopathies* were included).

The second step was to conduct a "broad" search to identify cases that might be rhabdomyolysis or myopathy but were not specifically recognized as such at the time they were reported. Such rhabdomyolysis- or myopathy-like cases were identified by searching for cases not specifically reporting events that coded to any of the PTs listed in Table A.2.a.1, but reporting events that coded to at least one of the 40 relevant PTs listed in Table A.2.a.2.

The searches of the company's safety database using the candidate SMQ identified a total of 251 cases for Compound 1 and 318 cases for Compound 2. The results of these searches are summarized in Table A.2.a.3, Table A.2.a.4 and Table A.2.a.5. A listing of the number of cases reporting each of the relevant MedDRA PTs is presented in Table A.2.a.3. The five most commonly reported PTs for both Compound 1 and Compound 2 were PT *Myalgia*, PT *Blood creatine phosphokinase increased*, PT *Muscle weakness*, PT *Rhabdomyolysis* and PT *Myopathy*.

The number of cases identified by the narrow search and the number of cases added after the broad search is presented in Table A.2.a.4. It should be noted that for Compound 1 the majority of cases were identified by the broad search, while for Compound 2 the majority of cases were identified by the narrow search.

In Table A.2.a.5 the cases are further characterized by the presence of other PTs reported in the same case. Other than PT *Rhabdomyolysis* or PT *Myopathy*, the two most commonly reported PTs for both Compound 1 and Compound 2 were PT *Myalgia* (160 and 72 cases respectively) and PT *Blood creatine phosphokinase increased* (74 and 61 cases respectively). A number of cases for the two test products reported both of these PTs in the same case, reported either PT *Myalgia* or PT *Blood creatine phosphokinase increased* along with another narrow-search or broad-search PT or with a non-search PT that is often associated with rhabdomyolysis or myopathy (such as fever, fatigue, nausea, increased aminotransferases or increased lactic dehydrogenase). A case was considered to be potentially rhabdomyolysis or myopathy if it listed PT *Rhabdomyolysis*, PT *Myopathy*, or at least one other narrow PT (i.e. PT *Myalgia*, PT *Myalgia aggravated*, PT *Polymyalgia* or PT *Blood creatine phosphokinase increased*) or any broad PT with at least one non-search PT associated with rhabdomyolysis or myopathy. Using these criteria, in 73 (29%) of the 251 cases the proposed SMQ identified for Compound 1 and in 247 (78%) of the 318 cases the proposed SMQ identified for Compound 2 would be considered potential cases of rhabdomyolysis or myopathy.

In the majority of the 178 cases for Compound 1 and 71 cases for Compound 2 that reported only one broad-search PT, the SMQ search PT was the only reported adverse event term for the case. In these instances, it was considered unlikely that the case contained sufficient information to determine if the reported broad PTs were possibly the result of rhabdomyolysis or myopathy.

• A.2.a.D. Summary and conclusions

MedDRA terms were reviewed to identify search terms for inclusion in an SMQ constructed to identify cases of potential rhabdomyolysis or myopathy. This review identified a total of 49 relevant PTs. The primary allocation for these 49 PTs has listed them under six SOCs, 12 HLGTs and 17 HLTs. These 49 PTs can be divided into terms for inclusion in a narrow search to identify cases specifically reported to involve rhabdomyolysis and/or myopathy or myopathy-related manifestations such as muscle necrosis, myoglobinaemia or myoglobinuria, and a broad search to identify cases not specifically reported as rhabdomyolysis or myopathy but reporting other musculoskeletal, renal, metabolic or laboratory PTs that might involve rhabdomyolysis or myopathy.

The candidate SMQ was tested against two products, both of which had rhabdomyolysis added to the product labelling during their post-marketing experience.

The results of these tests indicate that the candidate SMQ satisfactorily identified an adequate pool of cases to be reviewed to determine if an association exists with rhabdomyolysis or myopathy for either of the test products.

References:

1. Basic requirements for the use of terms for reporting adverse drug reactions (IV). Pharmacoepidemiol Drug Saf. 1993; 2:149–53.
2. Bankowski Z, Bruppacher R, Crusius I, Gallagher J, Kremer G, Venulet J, editors. Reporting adverse drug reactions: definitions of terms and criteria for their use. Geneva: CIOMS; 1999:16–7.
3. Poels PJE, Gabreëls FJM. Rhabdomyolysis: a review of the literature. Clin Neurol Neurosurg. 1993; 95:175–92.
4. Omar MA, Wilson JP, Cox TS. Rhabdomyolysis and HMG-CoA reductase inhibitors. Annals Pharmacother. 2001; 35:1096–107.
5. Prendergast BD, George CF. Drug-induced rhabdomyolysis – mechanisms and management. Postgrad Med J. 1993; 69:333–6.

Table A.2.a.1. SMQ *Rhabdomyolysis/myopathy*-related PTs for narrow search *

System Organ Class (SOC)	High Level Group Term (HLGT)	High Level Term (HLT)	Preferred Term (PT)
Musculoskeletal and connective tissue disorders	Muscle disorders	Myopathies	Muscle necrosis
			Myopathy
			Myopathy aggravated
			Myopathy toxic
			Rhabdomyolysis
		Muscle-related signs and symptoms NEC	Myoglobinaemia
Renal and urinary abnormalities	Urinary tract signs and symptoms	Urinary abnormalities	Myoglobinuria
Investigations	Musculoskeletal and soft tissues investigations (excl. enzyme tests)	Musculoskeletal and soft tissues tests NEC	Blood myoglobin increased
			Myoglobin urine present

* See also changes in the current SMQ version.

Table A.2.a.2. SMQ *Rhabdomyolysis/myopathy*-related PTs for broad search *

System Organ Class (SOC)	High Level Group Term (HLGT)	High Level Term (HLT)	Preferred Term (PT)
Musculoskeletal and connective tissue disorders	Muscle disorders	Muscle-related signs and symptoms NEC	Muscle haemorrhage
			Muscle fatigue
			Muscle disorder NOS
		Myopathies	Compartment syndrome
		Muscle pains	Myalgia
			Myalgia aggravated
			Myalgia intercostal
			Polymyalgia
			Polymyalgia aggravated
		Muscle weakness	Muscle weakness aggravated
			Muscle weakness NOS
	Musculoskeletal and connective tissue disorders NEC	Musculoskeletal and connective tissue signs and symptoms NEC	Musculoskeletal discomfort
			Musculoskeletal pain
			Musculoskeletal disorder NOS

System Organ Class (SOC)	High Level Group Term (HLGT)	High Level Term (HLT)	Preferred Term (PT)
Injury, poisoning and procedural complications	Injuries NEC	Muscle, tendon and ligament injuries	Muscle rupture
Investigations	Musculoskeletal and soft tissue investigations (excl. enzyme tests)	Musculoskeletal and soft tissue histopathology procedures	Biopsy muscle abnormal
	Neurological and special senses investigations	Neurologic diagnostic procedures	Electromyogram abnormal
	Renal and urinary tract investigations and urinalyses	Renal function analyses	Blood creatinine abnormal
			Blood creatinine increased
			Creatinine renal clearance decreased
			Glomerular filtration rate abnormal
			Glomerular filtration rate decreased
			Renal clearance NOS decreased
	Enzyme investigations NEC	Skeletal and cardiac muscle analyses	Blood creatine phosphokinase abnormal NOS
			Blood creatine phosphokinase increased
			Blood creatine phosphokinase MM increased
			Muscle enzyme increased
	Water, electrolyte and mineral investigations	Mineral and electrolyte analyses	Blood calcium decreased

System Organ Class (SOC)	High Level Group Term (HLGT)	High Level Term (HLT)	Preferred Term (PT)
Renal and urinary disorders	Renal disorders (excl. nephropathies)	Renal failure and impairment	Anuria
			Oliguria
			Progressive renal failure
			Renal failure acute
			Renal failure acute on chronic
			Renal failure aggravated
			Renal failure chronic aggravated
			Renal impairment NOS
		Renal vascular and ischaemic conditions	Renal tubular necrosis
	Urinary tract signs and symptoms	Urinary abnormalities	Chromaturia
Respiratory, thoracic and mediastinal disorders	Thoracic disorders (excl. lung and pleura)	Diaphragmatic disorders (excl. congenital)	Diaphragm muscle weakness
Metabolism and nutrition disorders	Bone, calcium, magnesium and phosphorus metabolism disorders	Calcium decreased disorders	Hypocalcaemia

* See also changes in the current SMQ version.

As MedDRA has been upversioned, the following changes have occurred (MedDRA version):

Addition of broad terms
   Myositis (v8.1).
   Creatinine renal clearance abnormal (v11.1).

Demotion to LLT
   Polymyalgia (under Myalgia, v9.1).

Table A.2.a.3. Health-care professional, nonclinical study cases reporting SMQ *Rhabdomyolysis/myopathy*-related MedDRA PTs for two test products reported to testing company's safety database during the time periods under review

Number of cases		
MedDRA PT	Compound 1	Compound 2
Blood myoglobin increased[A]	–	1
Muscle necrosis[A]	–	5

Number of cases		
Myoglobin urine present[A]	–	–
Myoglobinaemia[A]	–	–
Myoglobinuria[A]	–	3
Myopathy[A]	6	13
Myopathy aggravated[A]	–	–
Myopathy toxic[A]	–	–
Rhabdomyolysis[A]	14	189
Anuria[B]	–	–
Biopsy muscle abnormal[B]	–	–
Blood calcium decreased[B]	–	–
Blood creatine phosphokinase abnormal NOS[B]		
Blood creatine phosphokinase increased[B]		61
Blood creatine phosphokinase MM increased[B]	–	–
Blood creatinine abnormal[B]	–	–
Blood creatinine increased[B]	–	8
Chromaturia[B]	4	7
Compartment syndrome[B]	–	–
Creatinine renal clearance decreased[B]	–	–
Diaphragm muscle weakness[B]	–	–
Electromyogram abnormal[B]	–	–
Glomerular filtration rate abnormal[B]	–	–
Glomerular filtration rate decreased[B]	–	–
Hypocalcaemia[B]	–	–
Muscle disorder NOS[B]	–	–
Muscle enzyme increased[B]	–	–
Muscle fatigue[B]	1	–
Muscle haemorrhage[B]	–	–
Muscle rupture[B]	–	–
Muscle weakness aggravated[B]	–	2
Muscle weakness NOS[B]	11	20
Musculoskeletal discomfort[B]	–	1
Musculoskeletal disorder NOS[B]	–	–
Musculoskeletal pain[B]	1	1
Myalgia[B]	160	72
Myalgia aggravated[B]	1	–
Myalgia intercostal[B]	–	–
Oliguria[B]	–	–

Number of cases		
Polymyalgia[B]	1	–
Polymyalgia aggravated[B]	–	–
Progressive renal failure[B]	–	–
Renal clearance NOS decreased[B]	–	–
Renal failure acute[B]	1	13
Renal failure acute or chronic[B]	–	–
Renal failure aggravated[B]	–	–
Renal failure chronic aggravated[B]	–	–
Renal impairment NOS[B]	2	22
Renal tubular necrosis[B]	–	3
Total cases meeting any SMQ search criteria	**251**	**318**
Total health-care professional nonclinical study cases	**1716**	**822**

[A] Event term for inclusion in narrow search.
[B] Event term for inclusion in broad search.

Table A.2.a.4. Number of nonclinical study cases reported by health-care professionals identified by narrow and broad search for SMQ *Rhabdomyolysis/myopathy*-related events

Number of cases returned after each search		
Search type	Compound 1	Compound 2
Narrow search	30	213
Broad search[A]	221	105
Total cases meeting any SMQ search criteria	**251**	**318**
Total health-care professional nonclinical study cases	**1716**	**822**

[A] Cases reporting only broad search terms without reporting any narrow search terms.

Table A.2.a.5. Number of nonclinical study cases reported by health-care professionals identified by search for SMQ *Rhabdomyolysis/myopathy*-related events, further categorized by the presence of other PTs reported in the same case

Number of cases		
Search PTs categorized by presence of other reported PTs	Compound 1	Compound 2
Rhabdomyolysis and/or myopathy	20	201
Myalgia, myalgia aggravated, or polymyalgia and blood creatine phosphokinase increased	17	21
Myalgia, myalgia aggravated, or polymyalgia with at least one narrow PT other than rhabdomyolysis or myopathy	2	3

Number of cases		
Myalgia, myalgia aggravated, or polymyalgia with at least one additional broad PT[A]	1	–
Blood creatine phosphokinase increased with at least one narrow PT other than rhabdomyolysis or myopathy	–	4
Blood creatine phosphokinase increased with at least one additional broad PT[B]	–	1
Myalgia, myalgia aggravated, or polymyalgia with at least one non-search PT associated with rhabdomyolysis or myopathy	17	3
Blood creatine phosphokinase increased with at least one non-search PT associated with rhabdomyolysis or myopathy	6	2
Other narrow PT with at least one other broad PT	–	2
Other narrow PTs with at least one at least one non-search PT associated with rhabdomyolysis or myopathy	2	3
Other narrow PTs only relevant PT	8	7
Total cases of potential *Rhabdomyolysis* or *Myopathy*[C]	**73**	**247**
Myalgia, myalgia aggravated, or polymyalgia only relevant PT	122	40
Blood creatine phosphokinase increased only relevant PT	49	26
Other broad PTs only relevant PT	7	5
Total cases reporting only one broad PT	**178**	**71**
Total cases meeting any SMQ search criteria	**251**	**411**

[A] At least one additional broad PT other than PT *Blood creatine phosphokinase increased*.
[B] At least one additional broad PT other than PT *Myalgia*, PT *Myalgia aggravated*, or PT *Polymyalgia*.
[C] Any case reporting PT *Rhabdomyolysis*, PT *Myopathy*, or ≥1 other narrow PT; PT *Myalgia*, PT *Myalgia aggravated*, or PT *Polymyalgia* and PT *Blood creatine phosphokinase increased*; or any broad PT with ≥ 1 non-search term associated with rhabdomyolysis/myopathy considered a potential case of rhabdomyolysis or myopathy.

APPENDIX 2.b. Example of SMQ development: SMQ *Anaphylactic reaction*

• A.2.b.A. Definition and background

Anaphylactic reaction is an acute hypersensitivity reaction/allergic reaction of the immediate type, characterized by one or more of the following symptoms:

- skin: itching, erythema, urticarial, angioedema;
- respiratory system: laryngeal oedema or spasm, bronchospasm;
- cardiovascular system: hypotension.

In addition, the following symptoms may occur:

- gastrointestinal system: abdominal cramps, diarrhoea;
- neuropsychological: anxiety, agitation, loss of consciousness.

• A.2.b.B. Methodology

MedDRA v5.1 was used to build the original SMQ *Anaphylactic reaction* and was later updated to MedDRA v7.0 for Phase I testing.

Using a "top-down" and "bottom-up" search approach, lists were created by a large pharmaceutical company and a regulator capturing any terms, at the PT level, representing events which may be noted during anaphylaxis. In a spreadsheet format, the pharmaceutical company's list and the regulator's list were positioned alongside the MedDRA SSC list for anaphylaxis, and this three-column table was then systematically reviewed from top to bottom. Unanimous agreement for/against inclusion of each term was achieved by the group. An initial list of possible terms associated with anaphylactic reaction based on these decisions was then created.

From this group of PTs, an algorithm of PT search terms was created to increase the specificity for retrieving reports of anaphylactic reactions from the pharmaceutical company's MedDRA-coded database.

SMQ *Anaphylactic reaction* consists of three parts:

1. A **narrow search** containing PTs that represent core anaphylactic reaction terms.
2. A **broad search** that contains additional terms that are added to those included in the narrow search. These additional terms are signs and symptoms possibly indicative of anaphylactic reaction.
3. An **algorithmic approach** which combines a number of anaphylactic reaction symptoms in order to increase specificity.

At the time the SMQ was released into production (MedDRA v8.1), the following PTs were included in the search:

Narrow search
Anaphylactic reaction, Anaphylactic shock, Anaphylactoid reaction, Anaphylactoid shock, Circulatory collapse, Shock, Type I hypersensitivity.

Broad search

The **broad** search contains all narrow search terms (see above) as well as the following PTs:

Column A – (Upper airway/Respiratory)
Acute respiratory failure, Asthma, Bronchial oedema, Bronchospasm, Cardio-respiratory distress, Chest discomfort, Choking, Choking sensation, Cough, Dyspnoea exacerbated, Dyspnoea, Hoarseness, Hyperventilation, Laryngeal dyspnoea, Laryngeal oedema, Laryngospasm, Laryngotracheal oedema, Oedema mouth, Oropharyngeal spasm, Oropharyngeal swelling, Respiratory arrest, Respiratory distress, Respiratory failure, Reversible airways obstruction, Sensation of foreign body, Sneezing, Stridor, Swollen tongue, Throat tightness, Tongue oedema, Tracheal obstruction, Tracheal oedema, Wheezing.

Column B – (Angioedema/Urticaria/Pruritus/Flush)
Allergic oedema, Angioneurotic oedema, Erythema, Exanthem, Eye oedema, Eyelid oedema, Eye swelling, Face oedema, Fixed eruption, Flushing, Generalised erythema, Oedema, Periorbital oedema, Pruritus, Pruritus generalised, Rash erythematosus, Rash generalised, Rash, Rash pruritic, Skin swelling, Swelling face, Swelling, Urticaria generalised, Urticaria, Urticaria papular.

Column C – (Cardiovascular/Hypotension)
Blood pressure decreased, Blood pressure diastolic decreased, Blood pressure systolic decreased, Cardiac arrest, Cardio-respiratory arrest, Hypotension.

- ## A.2.b.C. Algorithmic approach

The **algorithmic approach** combines a number of anaphylactic reaction symptoms in order to increase specificity. A case must include one of the following:

a. a narrow term; OR

b. a term from Column A (Upper Airway/Respiratory) AND a term from Column B (Angioedema/Urticaria/Pruritus/Flush); OR

c. a term from Column C (Cardiovascular/Hypotension) AND [a term from Column A (Upper Airway/Respiratory) OR a term from Column B (Angioedema/Urticaria/Pruritus/Flush)].

- ## A.2.b.D. Results of testing

Testing using a regulatory database

The regulatory database used for testing contained domestic adverse event reports from 1965 to the time of testing (approximately 180 000 cases). Coding of adverse reactions was based on WHO-ART (1998, 3rd quarter). Data for three test products were recoded from WHO-ART terms to MedDRA v7.0 PTs.

Three products were chosen for testing this SMQ. Product 1 and Product 2 were labelled for anaphylactic reaction, and Product 3 did not list anaphylactic reaction in its labelling. Reports from 1 January 1998 to 1 January 2004 were used for testing.

Table A.2.b.1 displays the number of cases containing SMQ *Anaphylactic reaction* MedDRA PTs for the three test products from the regulatory database. Table A.2.b.2 summarizes the number of cases retrieved using the narrow search, broad search and algorithmic approaches.

The narrow search alone was not considered to be sufficiently comprehensive to detect a majority of relevant cases of anaphylactic reaction, as this search retrieved primarily diagnosed cases. After review of a cross-section of individual cases, it was determined that the broad search retrieved a large number of irrelevant cases – particularly cases listing one or two terms from Column B (Angioedema/Urticaria/Pruritus/

Flush) only (e.g. PT *Pruritus* or PT *Urticaria*; see Table A.2.b.2). These cases would not correspond with the internationally recognized definition of anaphylactic reaction.[1] Therefore, a combination of symptoms was included to optimize this SMQ. The algorithmic approach combines a number of anaphylactic reaction symptoms in order to increase specificity. Although the broad search was adequate for including a majority of anaphylactic reaction cases, the algorithmic approach retrieved the greatest number of clinically relevant cases while disregarding a number of irrelevant cases that the broad search retrieved.

Testing using a pharmaceutical company database

The pharmaceutical company's database contained case reports from 1980 onwards coded in MedDRA v7.0.

Three products were chosen for testing this SMQ. Product A and Product B were labelled for anaphylactic reaction and Product C was not labelled for anaphylactic reaction. Reports from 1 January 1980 to 1 January 2004 were used for testing.

Table A.2.b.3 displays the number of cases containing SMQ *Anaphylactic reaction* MedDRA PTs for three pharmaceutical company test products.

Table A.2.b.4 summarizes the number of cases retrieved using the narrow search, broad search and algorithmic approaches.

Similarly to the results from the regulatory database, the narrow search did not detect a majority of relevant cases of potential anaphylactic reaction as this search retrieved primarily diagnosed cases. With the broad search, a large number of irrelevant cases were retrieved – particularly cases listing one broad term and a wide variety of other terms not related to anaphylactic reaction (see Table A.2.b.4). Again, although the broad search was adequate for including a majority of anaphylactic reaction cases, the algorithmic approach retrieved the greatest number of clinically relevant cases while disregarding a number of irrelevant cases retrieved by the broad search.

• A.2.b.E. Summary and conclusions

Based on the level of specificity and sensitivity required for particular clinical safety situations, all three types of searches – narrow, broad and algorithmic – are adequate. According to the tests performed, there is no evidence that additional symptoms need to be included in one or more category of the proposed searches.

The main content changes are associated with new MedDRA versions since creation of the SMQ.

As a result of version changes from MedDRA v7.0 to v15.1, the following changes occurred in the SMQ:

- **PT additions**: Category A (narrow) – *Anaphylactic transfusion reaction, First use syndrome,* and *Kounis syndrome*; Category B – *Circumoral oedema, Cyanosis, Nasal obstruction, Tachypnoea,* and *Upper airway obstruction*; Category C – *Eye pruritus, Injection site urticaria, Lip oedema, Lip swelling,* and *Ocular hyperaemia*; Category D – *Diastolic hypotension*.

- **PT category changes**: broad-scope PT *Hypotension* changed category from B (*Upper Airway/Respiratory*) to D (*Cardiovascular/Hypotension*) in MedDRA v9.1 and broad scope PT *Cyanosis* changed category from C (*Angioedema/Urticaria/Pruritus/Flush*) to B (*Upper Airway/Respiratory*) in MedDRA v15.0.

- **PT demotions**: in MedDRA v9.1 broad-scope PT *Dyspnoea exacerbated* (Category B) was demoted and linked to broad-scope PT *Dyspnoea* (Category B) already included in the SMQ, and in MedDRA v10.0 broad-scope PT *Urticaria generalized* (Category C) was demoted and linked to broad-scope PT *Urticaria* (Category C) already included in this SMQ.

- **Other change**: LLT *Respiratory dyskinesia* from broad-scope PT *Dyspnoea* (Category B) was promoted to PT and made inactive in the SMQ in MedDRA v9.1.

Results tables

Table A.2.b.1. Post-marketing cases reporting anaphylactic reaction-related MedDRA PTs for three test products reported to the regulator from 1 January 1998 to 1 January 2004 (MedDRA v7.0)

		Number of cases		
MedDRA PT	Scope	Product 1 (N=308)	Product 2 (N=283)	Product 3 (N=60)
Anaphylactic reaction	narrow	1	11	0
Anaphylactic shock	narrow	0	2	0
Anaphylactoid reaction	narrow	0	2	0
Anaphylactoid shock	narrow	0	0	0
Circulatory collapse	narrow	0	1	0
Shock	narrow	0	0	0
Type I hypersensitivity	narrow	0	0	0
Column A – (Upper Airway/Respiratory)				
Acute respiratory failure	broad	0	0	0
Asthma	broad	1	1	0
Bronchial oedema	broad	0	0	0
Bronchospasm	broad	2	0	0
Cardio-respiratory distress	broad	0	0	0
Chest discomfort	broad	13	2	2
Choking	broad	4	1	0
Choking sensation	broad	0	0	0
Cough	broad	17	3	0
Dyspnoea exacerbated	broad	0	0	0
Dyspnoea	broad	22	17	2
Hoarseness	broad	1	1	0
Hyperventilation	broad	0	0	0
Laryngeal dyspnoea	broad	0	0	0
Laryngeal oedema	broad	1	1	0
Laryngospasm	broad	0	0	0
Laryngotracheal oedema	broad	0	0	0
Oedema mouth	broad	1	2	1
Oropharyngeal spasm	broad	0	0	0
Oropharyngeal swelling	broad	4	3	0
Respiratory arrest	broad	5	0	0
Respiratory distress	broad	0	1	0
Respiratory failure	broad	0	0	0

		Number of cases		
MedDRA PT	Scope	Product 1 (N=308)	Product 2 (N=283)	Product 3 (N=60)
Reversible airways obstruction	broad	0	0	0
Sensation of foreign body	broad	0	0	0
Sneezing	broad	17	0	0
Stridor	broad	1	0	0
Swollen tongue	broad	2	3	1
Throat tightness	broad	11	0	0
Tongue oedema	broad	2	2	0
Tracheal obstruction	broad	0	0	0
Tracheal oedema	broad	0	0	0
Wheezing	broad	5	1	1
Column B – (Angioedema/Urticaria/Pruritus/Flush)				
Allergic oedema	broad	0	0	0
Angioneurotic oedema	broad	0	3	1
Erythema	broad	19	6	6
Exanthem	broad	0	0	0
Eye oedema	broad	0	0	0
Eyelid oedema	broad	4	1	1
Eye swelling	broad	0	0	0
Face oedema	broad	3	9	2
Fixed eruption	broad	0	1	0
Flushing	broad	16	2	0
Generalised erythema	broad	0	0	0
Oedema	broad	0	3	1
Periorbital oedema	broad	8	0	0
Pruritus	broad	85	10	12
Pruritus generalised	broad	0	0	0
Rash erythematosus	broad	15	7	3
Rash generalised	broad	0	0	0
Rash	broad	20	15	3
Rash pruritic	broad	0	0	0
Skin swelling	broad	0	0	0
Swelling face	broad	9	4	0
Swelling	broad	2	1	0
Urticaria generalised	broad	0	0	0
Urticaria	broad	183	16	5

MedDRA PT	Scope	Number of cases		
		Product 1 (N=308)	Product 2 (N=283)	Product 3 (N=60)
Urticaria papular	broad	0	0	0
Column C – (Cardiovascular/Hypotension)				
Blood pressure decreased	broad	0	0	1
Blood pressure diastolic decreased	broad	0	0	0
Blood pressure systolic decreased	broad	0	0	0
Cardiac arrest	broad	3	1	0
Cardio-respiratory arrest	broad	0	0	0
Hypotension	broad	11	1	1

Table A.2.b.2. Summary of narrow search, broad search and algorithmic approach of post-marketing cases reporting anaphylactic reaction-related MedDRA PTs for three test products reported to the regulator from 1 January 1998 to 1 January 2004 (MedDRA v7.0)

MedDRA PT	Number of cases		
	Product 1	Product 2	Product 3
Number of cases using narrow search	1	16	0
Number of cases using narrow and broad search	285	64	23
Total number of terms in narrow and broad search	487	134	23
Number of terms from narrow column	1	16	0
Number of terms from column A (Upper Airway/Respiratory)	108	38	5
Number of terms from column B (Angioedema/Urticaria/Pruritus/Flush)	364	78	18
Number of terms from column C (Cardiovascular/Hypotension)	14	2	0
Algorithmic approach:			
Number of cases using narrow search	1	16	0
Number of cases presenting a term from Column A (Upper Airway/Respiratory) **AND** a term from Column B (Angioedema/Urticaria/Pruritus/Flush)	51	10	4
or			
Number of cases presenting a term from Column C (Cardiovascular/Hypotension) **AND** [a term from Column A (Upper Airway/Respiratory) **OR** a term from Column B (Angioedema/Urticaria/Pruritus/Flush)]			
Total number of cases using the algorithmic approach (non-duplicate totals)	52	26	4

Table A.2.b.3. Cases reporting anaphylactic reaction-related MedDRA PTs for three pharmaceutical company test products from 1 January 1980 to 1 January 2004 (MedDRA v7.0)

MedDRA PT	Scope	Product A (N=6924)	Product B (N=3931)	Product C (N=830)
Anaphylactic reaction	narrow	69	3	0
Anaphylactic shock	narrow	23	2	0
Anaphylactoid reaction	narrow	3	3	2
Anaphylactoid shock	narrow	0	0	0
Circulatory collapse	narrow	18	8	4
Shock	narrow	24	25	0
Type I hypersensitivity	narrow	0	0	0
Column A – (Upper Airway/Respiratory)				
Acute respiratory failure	broad	7	6	0
Asthma	broad	23	1	4
Bronchial oedema	broad	0	0	0
Bronchospasm	broad	19	4	0
Cardio-respiratory distress	broad	0	1	0
Chest discomfort	broad	20	0	42
Choking	broad	1	0	0
Choking sensation	broad	1	0	3
Cough	broad	36	15	3
Dyspnoea exacerbated	broad	2	2	0
Dyspnoea	broad	155	52	16
Hoarseness	broad	13	1	1
Hyperventilation	broad	3	0	1
Laryngeal dyspnoea	broad	0	0	0
Laryngeal oedema	broad	8	1	0
Laryngospasm	broad	0	0	0
Laryngotracheal oedema	broad	0	0	0
Oedema mouth	broad	3	0	1
Oropharyngeal spasm	broad	0	0	0
Oropharyngeal swelling	broad	9	0	0
Respiratory arrest	broad	19	30	0
Respiratory distress	broad	22	87	0
Respiratory failure	broad	108	307	0
Reversible airways obstruction	broad	0	0	0

APPENDIX 2. EXAMPLES OF SMQ DEVELOPMENT

| MedDRA PT | Scope | Number of cases |||
		Product A (N=6924)	Product B (N=3931)	Product C (N=830)
Sensation of foreign body	broad	0	0	0
Sneezing	broad	1	0	0
Stridor	broad	2	0	1
Swollen tongue	broad	14	0	2
Throat tightness	broad	9	0	28
Tongue oedema	broad	5	0	0
Tracheal obstruction	broad	0	0	0
Tracheal oedema	broad	0	1	0
Wheezing	broad	17	1	0
Column B – (Angioedema/Urticaria/Pruritus/Flush)				
Allergic oedema	broad	0	0	0
Angioneurotic oedema	broad	16	0	2
Erythema	broad	94	10	3
Exanthem	broad	42	1	1
Eye oedema	broad	3	0	1
Eyelid oedema	broad	0	0	0
Eye swelling	broad	7	0	1
Face oedema	broad	19	0	5
Fixed eruption	broad	0	0	0
Flushing	broad	129	5	5
Generalised erythema	broad	5	1	0
Oedema	broad	20	7	1
Periorbital oedema	broad	5	3	0
Pruritus	broad	180	1	7
Pruritus generalised	broad	22	0	0
Rash erythematosus	broad	34	5	0
Rash generalised	broad	25	2	0
Rash	broad	313	32	13
Rash pruritic	broad	23	1	0
Skin swelling	broad	1	0	0
Swelling face	broad	28	1	2
Swelling	broad	17	1	1
Urticaria generalised	broad	8	0	0
Urticaria	broad	96	1	12
Urticaria papular	broad	0	0	0

		Number of cases		
MedDRA PT	Scope	Product A (N=6924)	Product B (N=3931)	Product C (N=830)
Column C – (Cardiovascular/Hypotension)	broad			
Blood pressure decreased	broad	27	6	4
Blood pressure diastolic decreased	broad	0	0	0
Blood pressure systolic decreased	broad	6	0	0
Cardiac arrest	broad	51	63	0
Cardio-respiratory arrest	broad	15	47	1
Hypotension	broad	150	93	5

Table A.2.b.4. Summary of narrow search, broad search and algorithmic approach of cases reporting anaphylactic reaction-related MedDRA PTs for three test products reported to the pharmaceutical company from 1 January 1980 to 1 January 2004 (MedDRA v7.0)

	Number of cases		
MedDRA PT	Product A	Product B	Product C
Number of cases using narrow search	136	41	6
Number of cases using narrow and broad search	1431	704	139
Total number of terms in narrow and broad search	1973	827	172
Number of terms from narrow column	137	41	6
Number of terms from Column A (Upper Airway/Respiratory)	497	506	102
Number of terms from Column B (Angioedema/Urticaria/Pruritus/Flush)	1090	71	54
Number of terms from Column C (Cardiovascular/Hypotension)	249	209	10
Algorithmic approach:			
Number of cases using narrow search	136	41	6
Number of cases presenting a term from Column A (Upper Airway/Respiratory) **AND** a term from Column B (Angioedema/Urticaria/Pruritus/Flush) or Number of cases presenting a term from Column C (Cardiovascular/Hypotension) **AND** [a term from Column A (Upper Airway/Respiratory) **OR** a term from Column B (Angioedema/Urticaria/Pruritus/Flush)]	149	53	8
Total number of cases using algorithmic approach (non-duplicate totals)	285	94	14

References:

1. Reporting adverse drug reactions: definition of terms and criteria for their use. Geneva: CIOMS; 1999:124.

APPENDIX 2.c. Example of SMQ development: SMQ *Hepatic disorders*

• A.2.c.A. Introduction

SMQ *Hepatic disorders* is relatively complicated since it concerns events which relate to a whole biological organ system. SMQ *Hepatic disorders* consists of a series of sub-SMQs in a hierarchical relationship to one another on several levels.

It comprises:

▶ a comprehensive search of all terms possibly related to the liver, irrespective of whether or not they are potentially related to drug effects;

▶ sub-SMQs for specific liver-related topics; and

▶ two pre-designed combinations of sub-SMQs for potentially drug-related liver disorders (one comprehensive, and the other for severe events only).

MedDRA terms related to the liver

Terms concerning hepatic disorders and related conditions are present in the following 12 MedDRA System Organ Classes (listed in alphabetical order): *Congenital, familial and genetic disorders; Gastrointestinal disorders; General disorders and administration site conditions; Hepatobiliary disorders; Infections and infestations; Investigations; Metabolism and nutrition disorders; Neoplasms benign, malignant and unspecified (incl cysts and polyps); Nervous system disorders; Respiratory, thoracic and mediastinal disorders; Skin and subcutaneous tissue disorders; Surgical and medical procedures.*

• A.2.c.B. Overview of SMQ *Hepatic disorders*

The SMQ *Hepatic disorders* (level-1) consists of a series of sub-SMQs (levels 2 to 5) in a hierarchical relationship to one another (see Figure A.2.c.1).

Some of the sub-SMQs contain only PTs of narrow scope (e.g. in MedDRA v18.0: sub-SMQ *Liver neoplasms, benign (incl cysts and polyps)*; sub-SMQ *Liver tumours of unspecified malignancy*; sub-SMQ *Liver-related coagulation and bleeding disturbances*; sub-SMQ *Hepatic disorders specifically reported as alcohol-related*; sub-SMQ *Pregnancy-related hepatic disorders*); the other hepatic disorders sub-SMQs contain narrow and broad search terms.

Figure A.2.c.1. Graphical overview of SMQ *Hepatic disorders* (MedDRA v18.0) *

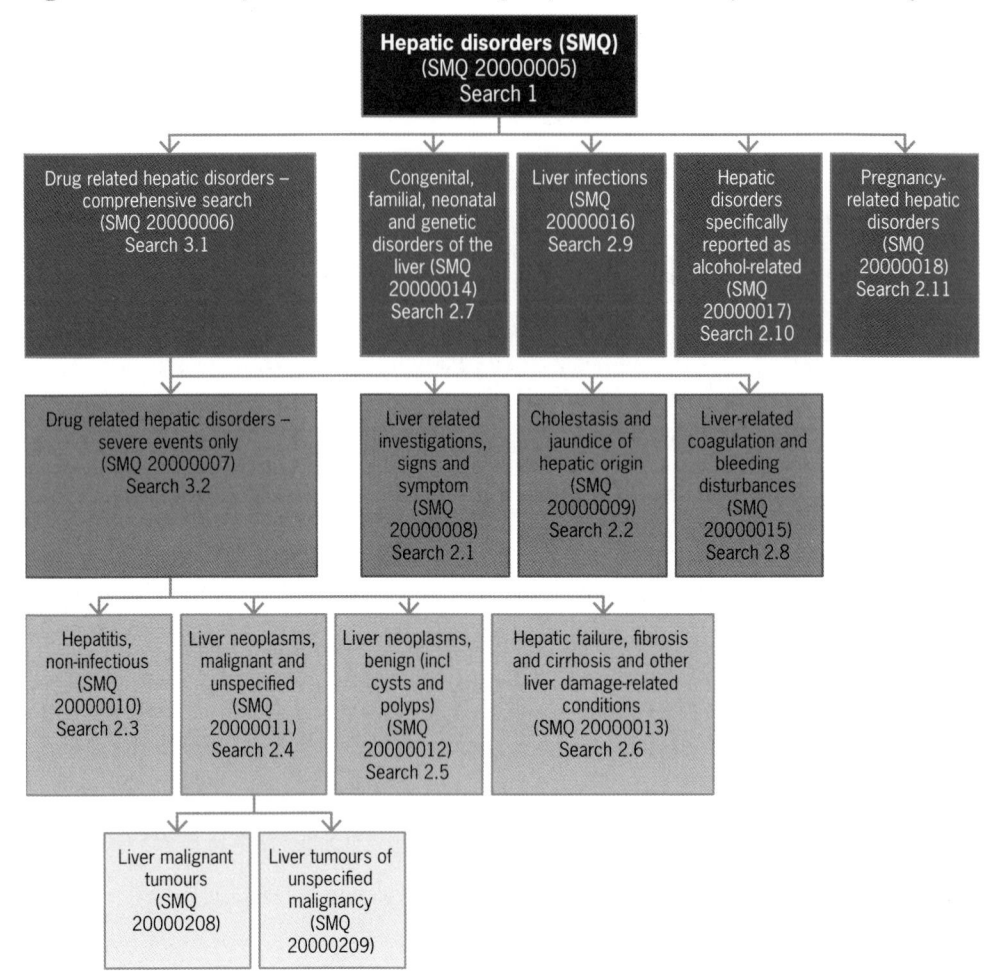

Hepatic disorders (SMQ)
(SMQ 20000005)
Search 1

- Drug related hepatic disorders – comprehensive search (SMQ 20000006) Search 3.1
- Congenital, familial, neonatal and genetic disorders of the liver (SMQ 20000014) Search 2.7
- Liver infections (SMQ 20000016) Search 2.9
- Hepatic disorders specifically reported as alcohol-related (SMQ 20000017) Search 2.10
- Pregnancy-related hepatic disorders (SMQ 20000018) Search 2.11

- Drug related hepatic disorders – severe events only (SMQ 20000007) Search 3.2
- Liver related investigations, signs and symptom (SMQ 20000008) Search 2.1
- Cholestasis and jaundice of hepatic origin (SMQ 20000009) Search 2.2
- Liver-related coagulation and bleeding disturbances (SMQ 20000015) Search 2.8

- Hepatitis, non-infectious (SMQ 20000010) Search 2.3
- Liver neoplasms, malignant and unspecified (SMQ 20000011) Search 2.4
- Liver neoplasms, benign (incl cysts and polyps) (SMQ 20000012) Search 2.5
- Hepatic failure, fibrosis and cirrhosis and other liver damage-related conditions (SMQ 20000013) Search 2.6

- Liver malignant tumours (SMQ 20000208)
- Liver tumours of unspecified malignancy (SMQ 20000209)

* This figure is valid for the MedDRA version given, but please see also the current MedDRA/SMQ version.

• A.2.c.C. Search strategy

There are three main types of search strategies with this SMQ.

An overview of all search strategies contemplated by the CIOMS WG is contained in Table A.2.c.1. Additional detail regarding the high-level strategies is provided following this table.

Table A.2.c.1. Summary topics of SMQ *Hepatic disorders* *

Search strategy	SMQ name	SMQ code
1	Hepatic disorders[A]	20000005
2.1	Liver related investigations, signs and symptoms	20000008
2.2	Cholestasis and jaundice of hepatic origin	20000009
2.3	Hepatitis, non-infectious	20000010
2.4	Liver neoplasms, malignant and unspecified	20000011
2.5	Liver neoplasms, benign (incl cysts and polyps)	20000012
2.6	Hepatic failure, fibrosis and cirrhosis and other liver damage-related conditions	20000013
2.7	Congenital, familial, neonatal and genetic disorders of the liver	20000014
2.8	Liver-related coagulation and bleeding disturbances	20000015
2.9	Liver infections	20000016
2.10	Hepatic disorders specifically reported as alcohol-related	20000017
2.11	Pregnancy-related hepatic disorders	20000018
3.1	Drug related hepatic disorders – comprehensive search	20000006
3.2	Drug related hepatic disorders – severe events only	20000007

[A] The numbering system 1–3.2 associated with each of the 14 search strategies listed in the table is agnostic and was created by the WG for clarity.
* See also changes in the current SMQ version.

Search strategy 1:

This search utilizes all of the terms in the entire SMQ *Hepatic disorders* and thus it is a comprehensive search on all types of events possibly related to the liver. It contains all MedDRA Preferred Terms concerning hepatic disorders and related conditions from the above-mentioned 12 MedDRA SOCs, and therefore retrieves all cases with liver-related conditions irrespective of whether or not they relate to drug-induced disorders.

This is a very broad general search on all hepatic disorders, including neoplasms, infections, congenital disorders, alcohol-related and pregnancy-related liver disorders, as well as all hepatitis terms, liver-related investigational terms, etc. The strategy includes the entire SMQ.

Search strategy 2:

This strategy utilizes one or more of the 11 component sub-SMQs. For ease of reference, the individual sub-SMQs are here referred to as searches 2.1–2.11. The individual sub-SMQs are designed to address a specific liver-related topic, and thus each is composed of a specific subset of liver-related terms (see more detail in the "Specifications" section below.) Since each sub-SMQ is designed to retrieve cases as specified by its topic, this strategy permits focused searches. Depending on the issue in question, a combination of several of these sub-SMQs may be appropriate, and some of the sub-SMQs are explicitly designed to be used in combination.

The sub-SMQs are not mutually exclusive and this fact must be taken into account when using combinations of them. Also, since a single Individual Case Safety Report may contain a number of different terms which could be included in different sub-SMQs, a given case may be retrieved by more than one sub-SMQ, so the recommended retrieval is by a combined "hit list".

Search strategy 3:

This strategy utilizes two pre-designed sub-SMQ search combinations specific to potential drug-related liver events. One combination is a comprehensive search, and the other is specific to severe drug-related hepatic disorders. Note that the hierarchical components of these two pre-designed search combinations are among the individual sub-SMQs discussed in search strategy 2.

Sub-SMQs by levels

Another way to describe the hierarchy for SMQ *Hepatic disorders* is to list all the levels of the sub-SMQs as they relate to each other.

The top, supraordinate, level-1 SMQ *Hepatic disorders* contains all the terms included in all of the subordinate hepatic disorders sub-SMQs.

At the next level (level-2 sub-SMQs), the terms are grouped into five level-2 stand-alone sub-SMQs. These represent "drug-related comprehensive search", "congenital", "liver infections", "alcohol-related" and "pregnancy-related" hepatic disorders (e.g. sub-SMQ *Drug related hepatic disorders – comprehensive search;* sub-SMQ *Congenital, familial, neonatal and genetic disorders of the liver;* sub-SMQ *Liver infections;* sub-SMQ *Hepatic disorders specifically reported as alcohol-related;* sub-SMQ *Pregnancy-related hepatic disorders*). Thus, sub-SMQ *Drug related hepatic disorders – comprehensive search* excludes events that are considered to be usually non-drug-related, such as "congenital", "liver infections", "alcohol-related" and "pregnancy-related" hepatic disorders.

Under sub-SMQ *Drug related hepatic disorders – comprehensive search* are the following four level-3 sub-SMQs: sub-SMQ *Drug related hepatic disorders – severe events only*, sub-SMQ *Liver related investigations, signs and symptoms*, sub-SMQ *Cholestasis and jaundice of hepatic origin* and sub-SMQ *Liver-related coagulation and bleeding disturbances.*

Further, sub-SMQ *Drug related hepatic disorders – severe events only* comprises four level-4 sub-SMQs: sub-SMQ *Hepatitis, non-infectious*, sub-SMQ *Liver neoplasms, benign (incl cysts and polyps)*, sub-SMQ *Liver neoplasms, malignant and unspecified*, and sub-SMQ *Hepatic failure, fibrosis and cirrhosis and other liver damage-related conditions.*

Finally, sub-SMQ *Liver neoplasms, malignant and unspecified* is divided into two level-5 sub-SMQs: sub-SMQ *Liver malignant tumours* and sub-SMQ *Liver tumours of unspecified malignancy.*

General remarks

In some instances it may be helpful to start with the full general search on the entire SMQ, while in other instances it may be better to exclude one or more of the specific sub-SMQs in order to eliminate conditions which are not applicable to a given question (e.g. liver infections or congenital and neonatal conditions).

Not included in this SMQ are terms solely associated with disorders of the gallbladder and the bile duct; there is another SMQ for this topic, SMQ *Biliary disorders.*

The term "hepatitis" is frequently misused in adverse reaction reporting by referring to any liver damage, whether or not histological lesions have been confirmed. This problem cannot, of course, be solved by an SMQ and requires an analysis of narratives and laboratory data fields in each ICRS.

Since this SMQ was released into production multiple modifications have been made to this SMQ (see Section A.2.c.F).

Note that all terms for supporting investigations, signs and symptoms are grouped only in sub-SMQ *Liver related investigations, signs and symptoms*. Thus, sub-SMQs of SMQ *Hepatic disorders*, which contain only diagnosis or only pathognomonic investigational results, are not independent queries. For example, to find all relevant cases of "liver infections", a search only by sub-SMQ *Liver infections* may be insufficient. Cases retrieved by terms for supporting investigational results, such as liver function tests (located in sub-SMQ *Liver related investigations, signs and symptoms*) may need to be included in order to retrieve a complete set of relevant cases; medical judgement should be applied.

As another example, sub-SMQ *Hepatic failure, fibrosis and cirrhosis and other liver damage-related conditions* is generally not intended to be used alone but in combination with sub-SMQ *Hepatitis non-infectious*.

• A.2.c.D. Specifications

A.2.c.D.i. Listing of the search strategies

Search strategy 1

▶ SMQ *Hepatic disorders*, SMQ code 20000005

General search contains all of the terms included in all hierarchical components of this SMQ. It is to be used for a comprehensive search retrieving all types of hepatic disorders. It combines all the terms in all the individual sub-SMQs 2.1 to 2.11.

Search strategy 2

This strategy covers 11 individual sub-SMQs on specific liver-related topics; for ease of reference, they are identified here as sub-searches 2.1-2.11:

▶ Search 2.1: sub-SMQ *Liver related investigations, signs and symptoms*; sub-SMQ code 20000008

▶ Search 2.2: sub-SMQ *Cholestasis and jaundice of hepatic origin*; sub-SMQ code 20000009

▶ Search 2.3: sub-SMQ *Hepatitis, non-infectious*; sub-SMQ code 20000010

▶ Search 2.4: sub-SMQ *Liver neoplasms, malignant and unspecified*; sub-SMQ code 20000011

▶ Search 2.5: sub-SMQ *Liver neoplasms, benign (incl cysts and polyps)*; sub-SMQ code 20000012

▶ Search 2.6: sub-SMQ *Hepatic failure, fibrosis and cirrhosis and other liver damage-related conditions*; sub-SMQ code 20000013

▶ Search 2.7: sub-SMQ *Congenital, familial, neonatal and genetic disorders of the liver*; sub-SMQ code 20000014

▶ Search 2.8: sub-SMQ *Liver-related coagulation and bleeding disturbances*; sub-SMQ code 20000015

▶ Search 2.9: sub-SMQ *Liver infections*; sub-SMQ code 20000016

▶ Search 2.10: sub-SMQ *Hepatic disorders specifically reported as alcohol-related*; sub-SMQ code 20000017

▶ Search 2.11: sub-SMQ *Pregnancy-related hepatic disorders*; sub-SMQ code 20000018

Search strategy 3

Strategy 3 involves searches for potential drug-related hepatic disorders, based on designed, pre-formed combinations of sub-SMQs.

▶ Search 3.1: sub-SMQ *Drug related hepatic disorders – comprehensive search*; sub-SMQ code 20000006

This sub-SMQ is a pre-designed combination of the following:

— Sub-SMQ *Drug related hepatic disorders – severe events only*;

— Sub-SMQ *Liver related investigations, signs and symptoms*;

— Sub-SMQ *Cholestasis and jaundice of hepatic origin*;

— Sub-SMQ *Liver-related coagulation and bleeding disturbances*.

▶ Search 3.2: sub-SMQ *Drug related hepatic disorders – severe events only*; sub-SMQ code 20000007

This sub-SMQ is a pre-designed combination of the following:

— Sub-SMQ *Hepatitis, non-infectious*;

— Sub-SMQ *Liver neoplasms, malignant and unspecified*;

— Sub-SMQ *Liver neoplasms, benign (incl cysts and polyps)*;

— Sub-SMQ *Hepatic failure, fibrosis and cirrhosis and other liver damage-related conditions*.

A.2.c.D.ii. PT content

SMQ *Hepatic disorders* was originally developed and tested with terms from MedDRA v6.1. The SMQ was released for user testing in MedDRA v8.0 and subsequently into full production in MedDRA v8.1.

The next section provides the list of PT terms in the initial SMQ using MedDRA v6.1, followed by the testing results which are also based on the initial SMQ designed in MedDRA v6.1. The PT terms are listed only by their primary SOC location, although many of the PTs also have secondary links to the SOC *Hepatobiliary disorders*. If a secondary link is given, this is indicated either in the text or as legend information. The same happens with MedDRA version change information.

Listing of PTs (both the PT content and sub-SMQ names reflect the initial MedDRA v6.1)

Search strategy 1: SMQ *Hepatic disorders* – General search

To be used for a general search retrieving all types of hepatic disorders. It combines all of the terms of the sub-SMQs (searches 2.1 to 2.11 listed in Table A.2.c.1).

Search strategy 2: Individual sub-SMQs for specific liver-related topics

Search 2.1: sub-SMQ *Liver related investigations, signs and symptoms*

Many of the terms of this sub-SMQ belong to the HLGT *Hepatobiliary investigations* of the SOC *Investigations*. Terms for laboratory test names (without indicating a result) or for investigations with a normal outcome are not included.

This search also contains all terms of the HLT *Hepatobiliary signs and symptoms* of the SOC *Hepatobiliary disorders*, and several PTs from other SOCs.

Included are:

▶ The following PTs from primary HLT *Liver function analyses*:

Alanine aminotransferase abnormal, Alanine aminotransferase increased, Ammonia abnormal, Ammonia increased, Aspartate aminotransferase abnormal, Aspartate aminotransferase increased, Bile output abnormal, Bile output decreased, Bilirubin conjugated increased, Blood bilirubin abnormal, Blood bilirubin increased, Blood bilirubin unconjugated increased, Blood cholinesterase abnormal, Blood cholinesterase decreased, Bromosulphthalein test abnormal, Galactose elimination capacity test abnormal, Galactose elimination capacity test decreased, Gamma-glutamyltransferase abnormal, Gamma-glutamyltransferase increased, Guanase increased, Hepaplastin abnormal, Hepaplastin decreased, Hepatic enzyme decreased, Hepatic enzyme increased, Hepatic enzyme abnormal, Hyperammonaemia, Leucine aminopeptidase increased, Liver function test abnormal, Retinol binding protein decreased, Transaminases abnormal, Transaminases increased, Urine bilirubin increased, Urobilin urine present, 5'nucleotidase increased.

▶ The following PT of the HLT *Hepatobiliary histopathology procedures*:

Biopsy liver abnormal.

- The following PTs of the HLT *Hepatobiliary imaging procedures*:

Liver scan abnormal, Ultrasound liver abnormal, X-ray hepatobiliary abnormal.

- The following PTs of the HLT *Tissue enzyme analyses NEC*:

Blood alkaline phosphatase increased, Blood alkaline phosphatase abnormal.

- The following PT of the HLT *Hepatic enzyme and function abnormalities*:

Hepatic function abnormal.

- The following PTs of the HLT *Hepatobiliary signs and symptoms*:

Caput medusae, Foetor hepaticus, Hepatic congestion, Hepatic pain, Hepatomegaly, Hepatosplenomegaly, Liver induration, Liver tenderness, Perihepatic discomfort.

- The following PT of the HLT *Hepatobiliary disorders NEC*:

Hypercholia.

- The following additional PTs:

Ascites, Haemorrhagic ascites, Kayser-Fleischer ring, Hyperbilirubinaemia, Hypoalbuminaemia, Liver palpable subcostal, Hepatic mass.

- The PT *Oedema due to hepatic disease* of the SOC *General disorders and administration site conditions*.

Search 2.2: sub-SMQ *Cholestasis and jaundice of hepatic origin*

This sub-SMQ includes all conditions associated with jaundice or cholestasis of possible hepatic origin and therefore excludes PTs indicating jaundice caused by haemolytic conditions, the PT *Jaundice extrahepatic obstructive* and the PT *Weil's disease* (with LLT *Hemorrhagic leptospirosis with jaundice*).

Included are:

- SOC *Hepatobiliary disorders*
  - HLT *Cholestasis and jaundice*:

PTs Cholestasis, Hepatitis cholestatic, Hyperbilirubinaemia, Jaundice cholestatic, Jaundice hepatocellular, Jaundice.

  - HLT *Hepatobiliary disorders NEC*:

PT Cholaemia.

  - HLT *Hepatic enzymes and function abnormalities*:

PT Bilirubin excretion disorder.

- SOC *Eye disorders*:

PT Ocular icterus.

- SOC *Investigations*
  - HLT *Liver function analyses*:

PT Icterus index increased.

Search 2.3: sub-SMQ *Hepatitis non-infectious*

Included PTs are from the SOC *Hepatobiliary disorders*.

- The following PTs of the HLT *Hepatocellular damage and hepatitis NEC*:

Autoimmune hepatitis, Chronic hepatitis, Cytolytic hepatitis, Hepatitis acute, Hepatitis chronic active, Hepatitis chronic persistent, Hepatitis fulminant, Hepatitis granulomatous, Hepatitis, Hepatitis toxic, Ischaemic hepatitis, Non-alcoholic steatohepatitis.

The remaining PTs of this HLT are included in searches 2.7 and 2.11 (see Table A.2.c.1).

- PT *Hepatitis cholestatic* of the HLT *Cholestasis and jaundice*.
- PT *Radiation hepatitis* of the HLT *Radiation injuries*.

Search 2.4: sub-SMQ *Liver neoplasms malignant and unspecified*

All terms of this search belong to the HLGT *Hepatobiliary neoplasms malignant and unspecified* of the SOC *Neoplasms benign, malignant and unspecified (incl cysts and polyps)*.

Included are:

- All PTs of the HLT *Hepatic neoplasms malignant*:

Hepatic cancer metastatic, Hepatic cancer stage I, Hepatic cancer stage II, Hepatic cancer stage III, Hepatic cancer stage IV, Hepatic neoplasm malignant non-resectable, Hepatic neoplasm malignant, Hepatic neoplasm malignant recurrent, Hepatic neoplasm malignant resectable, Liver carcinoma ruptured.

- Both PTs of the HLT *Hepatoblastomas*:

Hepatoblastoma, Hepatoblastoma recurrent.

- The following PTs of the HLT *Hepatobiliary neoplasms malignant NEC*:

Hepatobiliary carcinoma in situ, Malignant hepatobiliary neoplasm, Mixed hepatocellular cholangiocarcinoma.

- The following PTs of the HLT *Hepatobiliary neoplasms malignancy unspecified*:

Hepatic neoplasm, Hepatobiliary neoplasm.

Search 2.5: sub-SMQ *Liver neoplasms benign*

All terms of this search belong to the SOC *Neoplasms benign, malignant and unspecified (incl cysts and polyps)*. Included terms are from the HLGT *Hepatic and biliary neoplasms benign*.

- The following PTs of the HLT *Hepatobiliary neoplasms benign*:

Benign hepatic neoplasm, Focal nodular hyperplasia, Haemangioma of liver, Hepatic adenoma, Hepatic cyst, Hepatic cyst ruptured, Hepatic haemangioma rupture.

Search 2.6: sub-SMQ *Hepatic failure, fibrosis and cirrhosis and other liver damage-related conditions*

This sub-SMQ is, as a rule, not used alone but in combination with sub-SMQ *Hepatitis non-infectious*. Note that PT *Cardiac cirrhosis* is not included because it is secondary to a cardiac condition.

Included are:

- SOC *Hepatobiliary disorders*

— All PTs of the HLT *Hepatic failure and associated disorders*:

Hepatic failure, Hepatorenal failure, Hepatorenal syndrome.

— The following PTs of the HLT *Hepatic fibrosis and cirrhosis*:

Biliary cirrhosis, Hepatic cirrhosis, Biliary cirrhosis primary, Lupoid hepatic cirrhosis, Hepatic fibrosis, Biliary fibrosis, Nodular regenerative hyperplasia.

(PT *Cirrhosis alcoholic* is included in sub-search 2.10 and PT *Congenital hepatic fibrosis* is included in sub-search 2.7 [see Table A.2.c.1]).

- The following PTs of the HLT *Hepatocellular damage and hepatitis NEC*:

Hepatic necrosis, Hepatic steatosis, Hepatocellular damage, Hepatocellular foamy cell syndrome, Hepatotoxicity, Non-alcoholic steatohepatitis, Portal triaditis, Reye's syndrome.

- The following PTs of the HLT *Hepatic and hepatobiliary disorders NEC*:

Hepatobiliary disease, Liver disorder, Hepatic lesion, Hepatic atrophy.

- PT *Portal hypertension* of the HLT *Hepatic vascular disorders.*

▶ SOC *Nervous system disorders*

- PTs *Asterixis, Coma hepatic and Hepatic encephalopathy.*

▶ SOC *Gastrointestinal disorders*

- PTs *Ascites, Varices oesophageal, Oesophageal varices haemorrhage.*

▶ SOC *Skin and subcutaneous tissue disorders*

- PT *Spider naevus.*

▶ SOC *Respiratory, thoracic and mediastinal disorders*

- PT *Hepatopulmonary syndrome.*

▶ SOC *Surgical and medical procedures*

- PTs *Liver transplant, Liver and small intestine transplant, Renal and liver transplant, Hepatectomy, Liver operation.*

▶ SOC *General disorders and administration site conditions*

- PT *Oedema due to hepatic disease.*

Search 2.7: sub-SMQ *Congenital, familial, neonatal and genetic disorders of the liver*

Included are:

▶ SOC *Congenital, familial and genetic disorders*

- The following PTs of the HLT *Hepatobiliary abnormalities congenital*:

Accessory liver lobe, Alagille syndrome, Congenital absence of bile ducts, Congenital cystic disease of liver, Congenital hepatic fibrosis, Congenital hepatobiliary anomaly, Congenital hepatomegaly, Dilatation intrahepatic duct congenital, Hereditary haemochromatosis, Polycystic liver disease.

- The following PTs with a secondary link to the HLT *Hepatic metabolic disorders*:

Porphyria acute, Porphyria non-acute, Pseudoporphyria, Hepato-lenticular degeneration.

- The following PT with a secondary link to the HLT *Hepatic and hepatobiliary disorders NEC*:

Cerebrohepatorenal syndrome.

- The following PTs related to neonatal conditions:

Hepatosplenomegaly neonatal, Neonatal hepatomegaly, Hyperbilirubinaemia neonatal, Neonatal cholestasis, Jaundice neonatal, Kernicterus, Hepatitis neonatal, Hepatocellular damage neonatal.

Search 2.8: sub-SMQ *Possibly liver-related coagulation and bleeding disturbances*

This search includes decreases of coagulation factor levels which may be due to reduced liver function and changes in blood coagulation parameters depending on these factors.

Included are from the SOC Investigations:

▶ The following PTs of the HLT *Coagulation and bleeding analyses*:

Antithrombin III decreased, Blood fibrinogen abnormal, Blood fibrinogen decreased, Blood thrombin abnormal, Blood thrombin decreased, Blood thromboplastin abnormal, Blood thromboplastin decreased, Coagulation factor decreased, Coagulation factor IX level abnormal, Coagulation factor IX level decreased, Coagulation factor V level abnormal, Coagulation factor V level decreased, Coagulation factor VII level abnormal, Coagulation factor VII level decreased, Coagulation factor X level abnormal, Coagulation factor X level decreased, International normalised ratio abnormal, International normalised ratio decreased, Protein C decreased, Protein S abnormal, Protein S decreased, Prothrombin level abnormal, Prothrombin level decreased, Prothrombin time abnormal, Prothrombin time prolonged, Prothrombin time ratio abnormal, Prothrombin time ratio decreased, Thrombin time abnormal, Thrombin time prolonged.

Search 2.9: sub-SMQ *Liver infections*

Included are:

▶ SOC *Infections and infestations*

— All PTs of the HLT *Hepatitis viral infections*:

Hepatitis A, Hepatitis B, Hepatitis C, Hepatitis D, Hepatitis E, Hepatitis F, Hepatitis G, Hepatitis H, Hepatitis non-A non-B, Hepatitis non-A non-B non-C, Gianotti-Crosti syndrome.

— The following PTs of the HLT *Liver and spleen infections*:

Hepatobiliary infection, Hepatic infection, Hepatic cyst infection, Liver abscess, Portal pyaemia (splenic infections are not included).

— The following PTs linking to various infection related HLTs:

Hepatitis infectious mononucleosis, Hepatitis viral, Cytomegalovirus hepatitis, Hepatitis syphilitic, Hepatitis toxoplasmal, Hepatitis mumps, Hepatitis infectious, Viral hepatitis carrier, Adenoviral hepatitis, Hepatic candidiasis, Hepatosplenic candidiasis, Amoebic liver abscess, Hepatic echinococciasis, Schistosomiasis liver, Perihepatitis gonococcal, Weil's disease.

▶ SOC *Hepatobiliary disorders*

— The following PT of the HLT *Hepatic viral infections*:

Hepatitis post transfusion.

▶ SOC *Congenital, familial and genetic disorders*

— PT Congenital hepatitis B infection.

▶ SOC *Investigations*

— PTs: Anti-HBc antibody positive, Anti-HBe antibody positive, Anti-HBs antibody positive, Anti-HBc IgM antibody positive, Anti-HBc IgG antibody positive, Hepatitis A antibody positive, Hepatitis A positive, Hepatitis A antigen positive, Hepatitis A antibody abnormal, Hepatitis B positive, Hepatitis B antibody abnormal, Hepatitis B antibody positive, Hepatitis B DNA assay positive, Hepatitis B surface antigen positive Hepatitis B core antigen positive, Hepatitis B e antigen positive, Hepatitis C antibody positive, Hepatitis C positive, Hepatitis C RNA positive, Hepatitis D antibody positive, Hepatitis D antigen positive, Hepatitis D RNA positive, Hepatitis E antibody abnormal, Hepatitis E antibody positive, Hepatitis E antigen positive.

The following PTs of the SOC *Investigations* are **not included** in this search:

Hepatitis A virus, Hepatitis A screen, Hepatitis A antibody, Hepatitis A antigen normal, Hepatitis B virus, Hepatitis B antibody normal, Hepatitis B antibody negative, Hepatitis B antibody, Hepatitis B surface antigen negative, Hepatitis B surface antigen, Hepatitis B screen, Hepatitis B core antigen, Hepatitis B e antigen negative, Hepatitis B e antigen, Hepatitis B virus, Hepatitis C virus, Hepatitis C antibody, Hepatitis C antibody negative, Hepatitis C RNA, Hepatitis C RNA negative, Hepatitis C screen, Hepatitis D antigen,

Hepatitis D antigen negative, Hepatitis E antibody, Hepatitis E antibody normal, Hepatitis E antibody negative, Hepatitis viral test.

Search 2.10: sub-SMQ *Events specifically reported as alcohol-related*

This search contains terms specifically related to alcohol-associated disorders. These have not been included in any of the other sub-searches since alcohol-related terms are normally not searched for when looking for drug-induced liver injuries. Events that can be possibly alcohol-related but which also can have other causes (e.g. cirrhosis) have not been included here. Included PTs are:

▸ The following PTs of the HLT *Hepatocellular damage and hepatitis NEC*:

Alcoholic liver disease, Fatty liver alcoholic, Hepatitis alcoholic, Zieve syndrome.

▸ The following PT of the HLT *Hepatic fibrosis and cirrhosis*:

Cirrhosis alcoholic.

Search 2.11: sub-SMQ *Pregnancy-related hepatic disorders*

This search contains terms specifically related to pregnancy-associated disorders. These have not been included in any of the other hepatic sub-SMQs since they are normally not searched for when looking for drug-induced liver injuries, etc. Included PTs are:

▸ The following PT of the HLT *Cholestasis and jaundice*:

Cholestasis of pregnancy.

▸ The following PT of the HLT *Hepatocellular damage and hepatitis NEC*:

Acute fatty liver of pregnancy.

Search strategy 3: Searches with pre-designed combination sub-SMQs for possibly drug-related hepatic disorders

Searches 3.1 and 3.2 provide combinations of some of the searches 2.1 to 2.11 (see Table A.2.c.1) for terms associated with possibly drug-related hepatic disorders.

Search 3.1: sub-SMQ *Possibly drug related hepatic disorders – comprehensive search*

This broad, comprehensive search includes all terms (see Table A.2.c.1) from the following:

▸ Search 2.1: sub-SMQ *Liver related investigations, signs and symptoms*

▸ Search 2.2: sub-SMQ *Cholestasis and Jaundice of hepatic origin*

▸ Search 2.3: sub-SMQ *Hepatitis non-infectious*

▸ Search 2.4: sub-SMQ *Liver neoplasms malignant and unspecified*

▸ Search 2.5: sub-SMQ *Liver neoplasms benign*

▸ Search 2.6: sub-SMQ *Hepatic failure, fibrosis and cirrhosis and other liver related conditions*

▸ Search 2.8 sub-SMQ *Possibly liver related coagulation and bleeding disorders.*

Search 3.2: sub-SMQ *Possibly drug related hepatic disorders – severe events only*

This search is focused on severe, often serious reactions, and includes all terms (listed in Table A.2.c.1) from the following:

▸ Search 2.3: sub-SMQ *Hepatitis non-infectious*

▸ Search 2.4: sub-SMQ *Liver neoplasms malignant and unspecified*

▸ Search 2.5: sub-SMQ *Liver neoplasms benign*

▶ Search 2.6: sub-SMQ *Hepatic failure, fibrosis and cirrhosis and other liver damage-related condition.*

• A.2.c.E. Pre-release testing

The most important requirement for the quality of an SMQ is that it contains all the MedDRA terms to which cases relevant to the given question are coded. It is also important to avoid as far as possible nonspecific terms which, when reported alone without other more specific terms, are not suggestive of relevant cases for the topic of interest and thus increase background noise.

For the SMQ *Hepatic disorders* three approaches were chosen as follows.

A.2.c.E.i. Completeness of data – based on a regulatory authority database

Situation at the regulatory authority at time of testing

For the purpose of coding adverse reactions, WHO-ART was the terminology used at this regulatory authority until 2004. MedDRA implementation occurred in mid-2004, which was after the candidate SMQ testing. Therefore, the test was not directly run on MedDRA coded data; it was necessary to convert the data to be analysed using the MedDRA terminology.

Conversion of data

The code plan consisted of about 5700 non-English terms, considered as either translations of (4000) or assignments to (1700) terms of the original terminology. The non-English terms that were used for coding the ADRs were stored in the database in addition to the WHO-ART PT. ADR descriptions that were not reflected in WHO-ART were maintained verbatim in the database.

For the conversion to MedDRA v6.0, the links between the non-English terms and MedDRA were created on the basis of LLTs. Since MedDRA PTs are also LLTs, it was possible to use the existing PT translations to make an assignment at the LLT level. The conversion was done in four steps:

1. For terms with an exact string match to the respective MedDRA PT/LLT translation, no further review was considered necessary.
2. Terms with no exact string match to MedDRA but which were considered translations of WHO-ART terms were linked to LLTs according to the respective WHO-ART record number if included in MedDRA.
3. Remaining terms were reviewed and assigned to MedDRA LLTs on a term-by-term basis.
4. Verbatim terms that were not coded in WHO-ART were also reviewed term-by-term and linked to MedDRA LLTs where possible.

For the purpose of testing this candidate SMQ, it was possible to match all relevant terms with MedDRA v6.0.

Unlike other SMQs, the SMQ for hepatic disorders aims to include all liver-related terms and to reorder them in different sub-SMQs. Therefore, it can be anticipated that all cases describing liver-related conditions will be detected when using the full SMQ with all its subordinate levels. The test focused on detecting potential terms which were not yet covered in the sub-SMQs.

For the purpose of this test, case reports from a regulatory authority database from 1995 to 2004 were considered (approximately 89 000 cases). The SMQ PTs (all categories) were linked to database terms using the matches and assignments described above. Terms linked to one of the sub-SMQs were considered covered. All others were grouped and reviewed on the LLT level (about 7000) for potential relevance to this SMQ. The test showed that it was not necessary to include any additional terms.

A.2.c.E.ii. Testing of SMQ *Hepatic disorders* on pharmaceutical company A's database

Methods

In an effort to evaluate the two proposed predefined sub-SMQs for identifying potential cases of possibly drug-induced liver toxicity, a company drug safety database, coded in MedDRA v6.1, was searched using the proposed search strategies sub-SMQ *Possibly drug related hepatic disorders – comprehensive search* (search 3.1) and sub-SMQ *Possibly drug related hepatic disorders – severe events only* (search 3.2). The database contained cases of adverse events (serious and non-serious) reported spontaneously, including cases reported by health authorities and cases published in the medical literature. It also contained cases of serious adverse events reported from clinical studies and company-sponsored marketing programmes regardless of causality. It was reviewed for cases reported up to 18 February 2004 that contained a MedDRA PT belonging to the two candidate sub-SMQs, as an adverse event or co-manifestation, for four different compounds. Liver toxicity is attributed to two of the four drugs (Compound 1 and Compound 2) and is addressed in the company core data sheet for these two compounds. The remaining two compounds (Compound 3 and Compound 4) were not considered to be associated with liver toxicity at the time the query was tested.

Results and discussion

As a result of applying the two candidate sub-SMQs for possibly drug-induced hepatotoxicity to the data of the four test compounds in the database, a total of 32 PTs belonging to the search 3.2, which focuses on possibly severe events, were identified (see Table A.2.c.2). In addition, another 38 PTs that were not already contained in this search were retrieved with the broader, comprehensive events search of sub-SMQ 3.1. The results of the search for the four test compounds are summarized in Tables A.2.c.2 and A.2.c.3. In both tables bold figures indicate that the percentage of cases for a PT is higher for the test compounds than for all remaining drugs in the database (data for remaining drugs are not shown). A case having an adverse event/co-manifestation belonging to the "severe events only" sub-SMQ (search 3.2) may additionally contain another event/co-manifestation belonging to "comprehensive" sub-SMQ (search 3.1). It is also possible that a case contains more than one PT belonging to a sub-SMQ. In Table A.2.c.2, where PTs are displayed on an event/co-manifestation level, such a case can be counted more than once. On the other hand, in Table A.2.c.3, a case is counted only once because the data are displayed at case level. A listing of the number of each of the relevant MedDRA PTs reported with the four compounds is presented in Table A.2.c.2. The number of cases identified by the search for "severe events" (search 3.2) and the number of cases added after the broader "comprehensive" search (search 3.1) are presented in Table A.2.c.3. As the number of reports for each of the four compounds is quite different, percentages (number of reports of a certain PT belonging to the search reported for the compound in question, compared to the total number of events entered in the database for the compound in question) are also provided to ease the interpretation of the findings. Furthermore, the percentage figures of a PT reported for the four test compounds were compared to the percentage figure of that PT reported for all remaining compounds entered in the database (327 270 cases), and percentages with a higher frequency on a test compound compared to the remaining compounds are shown in bold. As can be seen from Table A.2.c.3, for the two products known to be associated with liver toxicity (Compounds 1 and 2), more than 10% of the total cases reported for each of these two compounds contain a PT belonging to one of these two candidate sub-SMQs (search 3.1 or 3.2). This is considerably more than for the other two compounds (Compounds 3 and 4) where it is 1.5% and 3.7%, respectively. As expected, compared to Compounds 3 and 4, the two compounds with known hepatotoxicity (Compounds 1 and 2) both have a higher percentage of events belonging to search 3.2 for "severe events" (1.5% and 3.6% vs. 0.4% and 1.9%) and for the "comprehensive" search 3.1 (11.0% and 6.4% vs. 1.1% and 2.1%). Thus, for products clearly associated with liver toxicity, the two proposed sub-SMQs seem to identify cases of possible liver toxicity adequately.

Summary and conclusions

Two candidate sub-SMQs (searches 3.1 and 3.2) of the liver SMQ, both specifically designed to identify possibly drug-induced liver toxicity, were tested in the company A drug safety database against four compounds, two of which were known to be associated with liver toxicity (positive test compounds), and two of which were not associated with liver toxicity (negative test compounds). The results of these tests indicated that the two proposed specific searches, sub-SMQ *Possibly drug related hepatic disorders – comprehensive search* and sub-SMQ *Possibly drug related hepatic disorders – severe events only,* seem to identify cases of drugs associated with liver toxicity – i.e. these two searches are an adequate tool to retrieve possibly relevant cases to assess if a drug has a hepatotoxic potential.

Table A.2.c.2. Adverse event and co-manifestation PTs belonging to the searches for possible drug-induced liver toxicity of four test products entered onto company A's drug safety database up to 19 February 2004, MedDRA v6.1

MedDRA PTs	Search	Search 3.1	Search 3.2	Compound 1 N	Compound 1 %	Compound 2 N	Compound 2 %	Compound 3 N	Compound 3 %	Compound 4 N	Compound 4 %
SMQ Search 3.2 (Only severe possibly drug-induced hepatic events)											
Autoimmune hepatitis	2.3	Y	Y	0	0.000%	0	0.000%	2	0.004%	0	0.000%
Cytolytic hepatitis	2.3	Y	Y	0	0.000%	12	**0.049%**	2	0.004%	1	0.008%
Hepatitis	2.3	Y	Y	8	0.186%	143	**0.578%**	35	0.070%	21	0.170%
Hepatitis acute	2.3	Y	Y	1	0.023%	3	0.012%	1	0.002%	0	0.000%
Hepatitis cholestatic	2.3	Y	Y	0	0.000%	73	**0.295%**	6	0.012%	5	0.041%
Hepatitis chronic active	2.3	Y	Y	0	0.000%	2	**0.008%**	0	0.000%	1	**0.008%**
Hepatitis fulminant	2.3	Y	Y	3	**0.070%**	4	0.016%	1	0.002%	1	0.008%
Hepatitis granulomatous	2.3	Y	Y	0	0.000%	4	**0.016%**	0	0.000%	0	0.000%
Hepatitis toxic	2.3	Y	Y	1	0.023%	15	**0.061%**	2	0.004%	1	0.008%
Total number of events in search 2.3	2.3			13	0.303%	256	1.035%	49	0.098%	30	0.243%
Hepatic neoplasm	2.4	Y	Y	1	**0.023%**	1	0.004%	0	0.000%	0	0.000%
Hepatic neoplasm malignant	2.4	Y	Y	1	0.023%	0	0.000%	4	0.008%	1	0.008%
Malignant hepatobiliary neoplasm	2.4	Y	Y	1	**0.023%**	0	-0.000%	1	**0.002%**	0	0.000%
Total number of events in search 2.4	2.4			3	0.070%	1	0.004%	5	0.010%	1	0.008%
Hepatic cyst	2.5	Y	Y	2	**0.047%**	0	0.000%	1	0.002%	0	0.000%
Total number of events in search 2.5	2.5			2	0.047%	0	0.000%	1	0.002%	0	0.000%
Ascites	2.6	Y	Y	4	0.093%	14	0.057%	5	0.010%	1	0.008%
Biliary cirrhosis	2.6	Y	Y	0	0.000%	0	0.000%	0	0.000%	1	**0.008%**

APPENDIX 2. EXAMPLES OF SMQ DEVELOPMENT

MedDRA PTs	Search	Search 3.1	Search 3.2	Compound 1 N	Compound 1 %	Compound 2 N	Compound 2 %	Compound 3 N	Compound 3 %	Compound 4 N	Compound 4 %
Coma hepatic	2.6	Y	Y	1	0.023%	1	0.004%	0	0.000%	2	0.016%
Hepatic atrophy	2.6	Y	Y	0	0.000%	0	0.000%	1	0.002%	0	0.000%
Hepatic cirrhosis	2.6	Y	Y	1	0.023%	3	0.012%	3	0.006%	3	0.024%
Hepatic encephalopathy	2.6	Y	Y	2	**0.047%**	6	0.024%	0	0.000%	1	0.008%
Hepatic failure	2.6	Y	Y	1	0.023%	32	0.129%	6	0.012%	4	0.032%
Hepatic fibrosis	2.6	Y	Y	0	0.000%	0	0.000%	0	0.000%	1	**0.008%**
Hepatic necrosis	2.6	Y	Y	3	**0.070%**	16	**0.065%**	2	0.004%	3	0.024%
Hepatic steatosis	2.6	Y	Y	3	**0.070%**	10	0.040%	21	0.042%	2	0.016%
Hepatocellular damage	2.6	Y	Y	0	0.000%	42	**0.170%**	6	0.012%	8	0.065%
Hepatorenal failure	2.6	Y	Y	0	0.000%	2	**0.008%**	0	0.000%	1	**0.008%**
Hepatorenal syndrome	2.6	Y	Y	0	0.000%	4	0.016%	0	0.000%	0	0.000%
Hepatotoxicity	2.6	Y	Y	0	0.000%	8	0.032%	1	0.002%	0	0.000%
Liver disorder	2.6	Y	Y	0	0.000%	24	0.097%	13	0.026%	6	0.049%
Oesophageal varices haemorrhage	2.6	Y	Y	0	0.000%	1	0.004%	0	0.000%	0	0.000%
Portal hypertension	2.6	Y	Y	0	0.000%	0	0.000%	1	0.002%	0	0.000%
Reye's syndrome	2.6	Y	Y	0	0.000%	2	**0.008%**	0	0.000%	0	0.000%
Varices oesophageal	2.6	Y	Y	0	0.000%	0	0.000%	1	0.002%	0	0.000%
Total number of events in search 2.6	2.6			15	0.350%	165	0.667%	60	0.120%	33	0.267%
SMQ Search 3.1 (comprehensive drug-induced hepatotoxicity search)[A]											
Alanine aminotransferase abnormal	2.1	Y		0	0.000%	0	0.000%	2	**0.004%**	0	0.000%
Alanine aminotransferase increased	2.1	Y		55	**1.282%**	105	0.424%	55	0.110%	25	0.203%
Ammonia increased	2.1	Y		1	**0.023%**	0	0.000%	0	0.000%	1	0.008%

APPENDIX 2. EXAMPLES OF SMQ DEVELOPMENT

MedDRA PTs	Search	Search 3.1	Search 3.2	Compound 1 N	Compound 1 %	Compound 2 N	Compound 2 %	Compound 3 N	Compound 3 %	Compound 4 N	Compound 4 %
Aspartate aminotransferase abnormal	2.1	Y		0	0.000%	0	0.000%	1	**0.002%**	0	0.000%
Aspartate aminotransferase increased	2.1	Y		57	**1.328%**	109	0.441%	48	0.096%	24	0.195%
Bilirubin conjugated increased	2.1	Y		3	**0.070%**	0	0.000%	2	0.004%	0	0.000%
Biopsy liver abnormal	2.1	Y		0	0.000%	1	**0.004%**	0	0.000%	0	0.000%
Blood alkaline phosphatase abnormal	2.1	Y		0	0.000%	1	0.004%	0	0.000%	0	0.000%
Blood alkaline phosphatase increased	2.1	Y		58	**1.352%**	108	**0.437%**	27	0.054%	14	0.113%
Blood bilirubin abnormal	2.1	Y		0	0.000%	0	0.000%	1	**0.002%**	0	0.000%
Blood bilirubin increased	2.1	Y		39	**0.909%**	71	0.287%	17	0.034%	12	0.097%
Blood cholinesterase decreased	2.1	Y		0	0.000%	0	0.000%	1	0.002%	0	0.000%
Gamma-glutamyl-transferase abnormal	2.1	Y		4	**0.093%**	0	0.000%	1	0.002%	0	0.000%
Gamma-glutamyl-transferase increased	2.1	Y		38	**0.886%**	55	0.222%	48	0.096%	20	0.162%
Hepatic congestion	2.1	Y		0	0.000%	0	0.000%	1	0.002%	0	0.000%
Hepatic enzyme increased	2.1	Y		58	**1.352%**	205	0.829%	96	0.192%	37	0.300%
Hepatic function abnormal	2.1	Y		2	0.047%	141	**0.570%**	14	0.028%	27	0.219%
Hepatic pain	2.1	Y		1	**0.023%**	3	0.012%	14	**0.028%**	0	0.000%
Hepatomegaly	2.1	Y		1	0.023%	23	**0.093%**	5	0.010%	6	0.049%
Hepatosplenomegaly	2.1	Y		0	0.000%	8	**0.032%**	3	0.006%	0	0.000%

APPENDIX 2. EXAMPLES OF SMQ DEVELOPMENT

MedDRA PTs	Search	Search 3.1	Search 3.2	Compound 1 N	Compound 1 %	Compound 2 N	Compound 2 %	Compound 3 N	Compound 3 %	Compound 4 N	Compound 4 %
Hypoalbuminaemia	2.1	Y		1	0.023%	7	0.028%	2	0.004%	0	0.000%
Liver function test abnormal	2.1	Y		10	0.233%	54	0.218%	40	0.080%	14	0.113%
Liver tenderness	2.1	Y		0	0.000%	0	0.000%	1	0.002%	0	0.000%
Urobilin urine present	2.1	Y		0	0.000%	0	0.000%	1	**0.002%**	0	0.000%
Total number of events in search 2.1	2.1			328	**7.644%**	891	3.602%	380	0.761%	180	1.459%
Cholestasis	2.2	Y		1	0.023%	51	**0.206%**	11	0.022%	4	0.032%
Hypoalbuminaemia	2.2	Y		0	0.000%	29	**0.117%**	1	0.002%	1	0.008%
Jaundice	2.2	Y		22	0.513%	223	**0.902%**	34	0.068%	26	0.211%
Jaundice cholestatic	2.2	Y		0	0.000%	30	**0.121%**	2	0.004%	4	0.032%
Ocular icterus	2.2	Y		2	**0.047%**	2	0.008%	3	0.006%	0	0.000%
Total number of events in search 2.2	2.2			25	0.583%	335	**1.354%**	51	0.102%	35	0.284%
Blood thromboplastin abnormal	2.8	Y		1	**0.023%**	0	0.000%	0	0.000%	0	0.000%
Coagulation factor decreased	2.8	Y		0	0.000%	0	0.000%	1	0.002%	0	0.000%
International normalised ratio abnormal	2.8	Y		0	0.000%	0	0.000%	2	**0.004%**	0	0.000%
International normalised ratio decreased	2.8	Y		0	0.000%	0	0.000%	6	**0.012%**	0	0.000%
Prothrombin level abnormal	2.8	Y		0	0.000%	0	0.000%	1	**0.002%**	0	0.000%
Prothrombin level decreased	2.8	Y		0	0.000%	12	**0.049%**	5	0.010%	1	0.008%
Prothrombin time abnormal	2.8	Y		0	0.000%	0	0.000%	1	0.002%	2	**0.016%**
Prothrombin time prolonged	2.8	Y		3	0.070%	18	0.073%	13	0.026%	2	0.016%
Prothrombin time ratio decreased	2.8	Y		0	0.000%	1	**0.004%**	0	0.000%	0	0.000%

MedDRA PTs	Search 2.8	Search 3.1	Search 3.2	Compound 1 N	Compound 1 %	Compound 2 N	Compound 2 %	Compound 3 N	Compound 3 %	Compound 4 N	Compound 4 %
Total number of events in search 2.8	2.8			4	0.093%	31	0.125%	29	0.058%	5	0.041%
Number of adverse events and co-manifestations belonging to search 3.1 and/or 3.2 reported with each drug				390	**9.089%**	1679	**6.788%**	575	1.152%	284	2.202%
Total number of adverse events and co-manifestations reported with each drug				4291	100%	24 735	100%	49 905	100%	12 339	100%

[A] Sub-searches from search 3.1 (comprehensive drug-induced liver toxicity search) that are not included in search 3.2 (severe drug-induced liver toxicity search).

Table A.2.c.3. Cases identified by searches 3.1 and 3.2

SMQ searches	Compound 1 N cases	Compound 1 % cases	Compound 2 N cases	Compound 2 % cases	Compound 3 N cases	Compound 3 % cases	Compound 4 N cases	Compound 4 % cases
Search 3.2 (search for severe drug induced liver toxicity)	26	1.52%	394	**3.57%**	101	0.40%	57	1.00%
Search 3.1[A] (broad search for drug-induced liver toxicity)	188	**11.03%**	702	**6.36%**	278	1.09%	120	2.11%
Number of cases containing a PT belonging to search 3.1 and/or 3.2[B]	214	**12.55%**	1106	**10.02%**	385	1.51%	210	3.70%
Total cases reported with each drug	1705	100.00%	11038	100.00%	25 536	100.00%	5675	100.00%

[A] Cases that included only terms from the comprehensive drug-induced liver toxicity search (search 3.1) without any terms from the severe liver toxicity search (search 3.2).
[B] Each case was counted only once, regardless of whether or not more than one PT belongs to the sub-SMQ.

A.2.c.E.iii. Testing of SMQ *Hepatic disorders* on pharmaceutical company B's database

A complementary analysis was used on the database of pharmaceutical company B and was also coded using MedDRA v6.1. Five compounds were analysed, two with known liver toxicity (Compound A, Compound B) and three with no known liver toxicity (Compound C, Compound D, Compound E). For all of the searches 2.1 to 2.11, odds ratios were calculated compared to the relative occurrence for the given term in the whole database.

Table A.2.c.4 shows the odds ratios for the percentage of events retrieved for the five drugs compared to that of all drugs available in the whole database for those sub-searches relevant for potential drug-related liver disorders.

Table A.2.c.4. Odds ratios calculated for percentage of events of possible drug-related liver toxicity searches for five test compounds compared to the entire database, MedDRA v6.1

Search/sub-SMQ	Compound A	Compound B	Compound C	Compound D	Compound E
1 Hepatic disorders	4.0	1.4	0.8	0.3	0.6
2.1 Liver related investigations, signs and symptoms	4.8	1.7	1.0	0.3	0.6
2.2 Cholestasis and jaundice of hepatic origin	2.6	1.1	0.3	0.2	0.6
2.3 Hepatitis, non-infectious	3.1	0.7	0.4	0.2	0.8
2.6 Hepatic failure, fibrosis and cirrhosis and other liver damage-related conditions	2.9	3.2	0.4	0.2	0.1
2.8 Liver-related coagulation and bleeding disturbances	1.9	1.3	0.2	0.3	0.5
3.1 Possibly drug related hepatic disorders – comprehensive search	4.0	1.4	0.8	0.3	0.6
3.2 Possibly drug related hepatic disorders – severe events only	3.0	2.0	0.4	0.3	0.4

The data show that, for all compounds for which no liver-related events were listed in the company core data sheet (Compounds C, D and E) the odds ratio was less than 1 for all of the searches/sub-SMQs, whereas for Compound A and Compound B it was greater than 1 for all except search 2.3 for Compound B. The odds ratios for Compound B were, for most searches, lower than for Compound A, which was in accordance with knowledge about these drugs when testing was performed.

- ## A.2.c.F. Modifications of SMQ *Hepatic disorders* over time

SMQ *Hepatic disorders* was released into full production in MedDRA v8.1. Since this SMQ was released into production there were multiple refinements over the years (for instance, as a result of MedDRA subscriber requests, periodic reviews of the SMQ, and regular incorporation of applicable new MedDRA PTs as a consequence of the release of new versions of the MedDRA dictionary). Changes have been implemented in both the SMQ hierarchy and its PT content. Future MedDRA releases will continue to incorporate new changes, as applicable.

A.2.c.F.i. Changes in the hierarchy of SMQ *Hepatic disorders*

Multiple changes have been implemented in the hierarchy of the SMQ *Hepatic disorders*: several sub-SMQs were renamed, several sub-SMQs changed scope, two level-5 sub-SMQs were added. Data documenting these changes were obtained from the *Introductory guide: SMQ version 18.0*[1] and copied below, listing the most recent change first:

In MedDRA v14.1, sub-SMQ *Events specifically reported as alcohol-related* was renamed to *Hepatic disorders specifically reported as alcohol-related,* representing a more precise description.

In MedDRA v14.0, two new sub-SMQs were added to existing sub-SMQ *Liver neoplasms, malignant and unspecified* to allow users to retrieve malignant-only events/cases, or events/cases of neoplasms of unspecified malignancy, or a combination of malignant and unspecified neoplasm events/cases. These two sub-SMQs are: *Liver malignant tumours* and *Liver tumours of unspecified malignancy.*

In MedDRA v12.1, a number of sub-SMQs were renamed (see Table A.2.c.5).

Table A.2.c.5. Renaming within SMQ *Hepatic disorders* *

Former sub-SMQ Name in MedDRA v12.0	New sub-SMQ Name in MedDRA v12.1
Possible drug related hepatic disorders – comprehensive search	Drug related hepatic disorders – comprehensive search
Possible drug related hepatic disorders – severe events only	Drug related hepatic disorders – severe events only
Liver neoplasms, benign	Liver neoplasms, benign (incl cysts and polyps)
Possible liver-related coagulation and bleeding disturbances	Liver-related coagulation and bleeding disturbances

* See also changes in the current SMQ version.

In MedDRA v12.1, the following sub-SMQs were modified in scope to include both broad and narrow search terms (formerly included only broad terms):

- Sub-SMQ *Cholestasis and jaundice of hepatic origin*
- Sub-SMQ *Congenital, familial, neonatal and genetic disorders of the liver*
- Sub-SMQ *Hepatic failure, fibrosis and cirrhosis and other liver damage-related conditions*
- Sub-SMQ *Hepatitis, non-infectious*
- Sub-SMQ *Liver infections*
- Sub-SMQ *Liver related investigations, signs and symptoms.*

In MedDRA v12.1, the following sub-SMQs were modified in scope to include narrow search terms (formerly included only broad terms):

- Sub-SMQ *Hepatic disorders specifically reported as alcohol-related*
- Sub-SMQ *Liver neoplasms, benign (incl cysts and polyps)*
- Sub-SMQ *Liver neoplasms, malignant and unspecified*
- Sub-SMQ *Liver-related coagulation and bleeding disturbances*
- Sub-SMQ *Pregnancy-related hepatic disorders.*

A.2.c.F.ii. Changes in the PT content of SMQ *Hepatic disorders*

Numerous PT changes have been implemented in the SMQ *Hepatic disorders* since its initial release. In general, PTs can be added to an SMQ, deleted from an SMQ, there can be a change in the PT content mapped to the narrow or broad scope of an SMQ, and finally there can be a status change where a PT is flagged as inactive. Changes at the SMQ PT level can occur independently or can be the consequence of an SMQ hierarchy change (e.g. change in the scope of a sub-SMQ, subdivision of an existing sub-SMQ into additional sub-SMQs, etc.). Complete data on the PT changes in SMQ *Hepatic disorders* can be obtained using the MSSO MVAT. Table A.2.c.6 includes several examples from this output.

Table A.2.c.6. Examples of PT changes in SMQ *Hepatic disorders* from initial publication to MedDRA v18.0 *

Change Type	SMQ Code	Sub-SMQ	PT	8.1 Status	18.0 Status	8.1 Scope	18.0 Scope
Added	20000008	Liver related investigations, signs and symptoms	Glutamate dehydrogenase increased				
Added	20000009	Cholestasis and jaundice of hepatic origin	Drug-induced liver injury				
Added	20000010	Hepatitis, non-infectious	Non-alcoholic steatohepatitis				
Added	20000013	Hepatic failure, fibrosis and cirrhosis and other liver damage-related conditions	Portal hypertensive gastropathy				
Added	20000208	Liver malignant tumours	Hepatic cancer stage I				
Added	20000208	Liver malignant tumours	Hepatic cancer stage II				
Scope Change	20000008	Liver related investigations, signs and symptoms	Liver function test abnormal			broad	narrow
Scope Change	20000008	Liver related investigations, signs and symptoms	Liver palpable			broad	narrow
Scope Change	20000013	Hepatic failure, fibrosis and cirrhosis and other liver damage-related conditions	Ascites			broad	narrow

Change Type	SMQ Code	Sub-SMQ	PT	8.1 Status	18.0 Status	8.1 Scope	18.0 Scope
Scope Change	20000015	Liver-related coagulation and bleeding disturbances	Coagulation factor IX level decreased			broad	narrow
Status Change	20000015	Liver-related coagulation and bleeding disturbances	International normalised ratio decreased	Active	Inactive		
Status Change	20000015	Liver-related coagulation and bleeding disturbances	Prothrombin time ratio decreased	Active	Inactive		
Deleted	20000011	Liver neoplasms, malignant and unspecified	Hepatic cancer stage I				
Deleted	20000011	Liver neoplasms, malignant and unspecified	Hepatic cancer stage II				

* See also changes in the current SMQ version.

As MedDRA versions evolve over time, it is always important to ensure that the MedDRA versions of the coded data and of the applied SMQ are one and the same version.

- ## A.2.c.G. Tabulation of PTs listed for SMQ *Hepatic disorders* MedDRA v8.0 and v18.0

PTs are listed in alphabetical order in the multi-part Table A.2.c.7 that follows.

Search 1: SMQ code 20000005
SMQ *Hepatic disorders*

This SMQ includes all terms of sub-searches 2.1 to 2.11 which are found in the tables below.

Search 2

Table A.2.c.7. Tabulation of PTs listed for SMQ *Hepatic disorders*, MedDRA v8.0 and v18.0 *

Search 2.1: SMQ code 20000008 *
Sub-SMQ *Liver related investigations, signs and symptoms*

Sub-SMQ Liver related investigations, signs and symptoms MedDRA v8.0	Sub-SMQ Liver related investigations, signs and symptoms MedDRA v18.0
5'nucleotidase increased	5'nucleotidase increased
Alanine aminotransferase abnormal	Alanine aminotransferase abnormal
Alanine aminotransferase increased	Alanine aminotransferase increased
Ammonia abnormal	Ammonia abnormal
Ammonia increased	Ammonia increased
Ascites	Ascites
Aspartate aminotransferase abnormal	Aspartate aminotransferase abnormal
Aspartate aminotransferase increased	Aspartate aminotransferase increased
	Bacterascites
Bile output abnormal	Bile output abnormal
Bile output decreased	Bile output decreased
	Biliary ascites
	Bilirubin conjugated abnormal
Bilirubin conjugated increased	Bilirubin conjugated increased
Biopsy liver abnormal	Biopsy liver abnormal
Blood alkaline phosphatase abnormal	Blood alkaline phosphatase abnormal
Blood alkaline phosphatase increased	Blood alkaline phosphatase increased
Blood bilirubin abnormal	Blood bilirubin abnormal
Blood bilirubin increased	Blood bilirubin increased
Blood bilirubin unconjugated increased	Blood bilirubin unconjugated increased
Blood cholinesterase abnormal	Blood cholinesterase abnormal
Blood cholinesterase decreased	Blood cholinesterase decreased
Bromosulphthalein test abnormal	Bromosulphthalein test abnormal
Caput medusae	
	Child-Pugh-Turcotte score increased
	Computerized tomogram liver
	Deficiency of bile secretion
Foetor hepaticus	Foetor hepaticus
Galactose elimination capacity test abnormal	Galactose elimination capacity test abnormal
Galactose elimination capacity test decreased	Galactose elimination capacity test decreased

Sub-SMQ Liver related investigations, signs and symptoms MedDRA v8.0	Sub-SMQ Liver related investigations, signs and symptoms MedDRA v18.0
Gamma-glutamyltransferase abnormal	Gamma-glutamyltransferase abnormal
Gamma-glutamyltransferase increased	Gamma-glutamyltransferase increased
	Glutamate dehydrogenase increased
Guanase increased	Guanase increased
Haemorrhagic ascites	Haemorrhagic ascites
Hepaplastin abnormal	Hepaplastin abnormal
Hepaplastin decreased	Hepaplastin decreased
	Hepatic artery flow decreased
Hepatic congestion	Hepatic congestion
Hepatic enzyme abnormal	Hepatic enzyme abnormal
Hepatic enzyme decreased	Hepatic enzyme decreased
Hepatic enzyme increased	Hepatic enzyme increased
	Hepatic fibrosis marker abnormal
	Hepatic fibrosis marker increased
Hepatic function abnormal	Hepatic function abnormal
	Hepatic hydrothorax
	Hepatic hypertrophy
Hepatic mass	Hepatic mass
Hepatic pain	Hepatic pain
	Hepatic sequestration
	Hepatic vascular resistance increased
	Hepatobiliary scan abnormal
Hepatomegaly	Hepatomegaly
Hepatosplenomegaly	Hepatosplenomegaly
Hyperammonaemia	Hyperammonaemia
Hyperbilirubinaemia	Hyperbilirubinaemia
Hypercholia	Hypercholia
	Hypertransaminasaemia
Hypoalbuminaemia	Hypoalbuminaemia
Kayser-Fleischer ring	Kayser-Fleischer ring
Leucine aminopeptidase increased	Leucine aminopeptidase increased
Liver function test abnormal	Liver function test abnormal
Liver induration	Liver induration
Liver palpable subcostal	
	Liver iron concentration abnormal
	Liver iron concentration increased

APPENDIX 2. EXAMPLES OF SMQ DEVELOPMENT

Sub-SMQ Liver related investigations, signs and symptoms MedDRA v8.0	Sub-SMQ Liver related investigations, signs and symptoms MedDRA v18.0
	Liver palpable
Liver scan abnormal	Liver scan abnormal
Liver tenderness	Liver tenderness
	Mitochondrial aspartate aminotransferase increased
	Molar ratio of total branched-chain amino acid to tyrosine
Oedema due to hepatic disease	Oedema due to hepatic disease
Perihepatic discomfort	Perihepatic discomfort
	Periportal oedema
	Peritoneal fluid protein abnormal
	Peritoneal fluid protein decreased
	Peritoneal fluid protein increased
	Pneumobilia
	Portal vein flow decreased
	Portal vein pressure increased
Retinol binding protein decreased	Retinol binding protein decreased
	Retrograde portal vein flow
	Total bile acids increased
Transaminases abnormal	Transaminases abnormal
Transaminases increased	Transaminases increased
Ultrasound liver abnormal	Ultrasound liver abnormal
Urine bilirubin increased	Urine bilirubin increased
Urobilin urine present	
	Urobilinogen urine decreased
	Urobilinogen urine increased
X-ray hepatobiliary abnormal	X-ray hepatobiliary abnormal

* See also changes in the current SMQ version.

Search 2.2: SMQ code 20000009 *
Sub-SMQ *Cholestasis and jaundice of hepatic origin*

Sub-SMQ Cholestasis and jaundice of hepatic origin MedDRA v8.0	Sub-SMQ Cholestasis and jaundice of hepatic origin MedDRA v18.0
Bilirubin excretion disorder	Bilirubin excretion disorder
Cholaemia	Cholaemia
Cholestasis	Cholestasis

Sub-SMQ Cholestasis and jaundice of hepatic origin MedDRA v8.0	Sub-SMQ Cholestasis and jaundice of hepatic origin MedDRA v18.0
	Cholestatic liver injury
	Cholestatic pruritus
	Deficiency of bile secretion
	Drug-induced liver injury
Hepatitis cholestatic	Hepatitis cholestatic
Hyperbilirubinaemia	Hyperbilirubinaemia
Icterus index increased	Icterus index increased
Jaundice	Jaundice
Jaundice cholestatic	Jaundice cholestatic
Jaundice hepatocellular	Jaundice hepatocellular
	Mixed liver injury
Ocular icterus	Ocular icterus
	Parenteral nutrition associated liver disease
	Yellow skin

* See also changes in the current SMQ version.

Search 2.3: SMQ code 20000010 *
Sub-SMQ *Hepatitis non-infectious*

Sub-SMQ Hepatitis non-infectious MedDRA v8.0	Sub-SMQ Hepatitis non-infectious MedDRA v18.0
	Acute graft versus host disease in liver
	Allergic hepatitis
Autoimmune hepatitis	Autoimmune hepatitis
	Chronic graft versus host disease in liver
Chronic hepatitis	Chronic hepatitis
Cytolytic hepatitis	
	Graft versus host disease in liver
	Granulomatous liver disease
Hepatitis	Hepatitis
Hepatitis acute	Hepatitis acute
Hepatitis cholestatic	Hepatitis cholestatic
Hepatitis chronic active	Hepatitis chronic active
Hepatitis chronic persistent	Hepatitis chronic persistent
Hepatitis fulminant	Hepatitis fulminant
Hepatitis granulomatous	
Hepatitis toxic	Hepatitis toxic

Sub-SMQ Hepatitis non-infectious MedDRA v8.0	Sub-SMQ Hepatitis non-infectious MedDRA v18.0
Ischaemic hepatitis	Ischaemic hepatitis
	Liver sarcoidosis
	Lupus hepatitis
Non-alcoholic steatohepatitis	Non-alcoholic steatohepatitis
	Portal tract inflammation
Radiation hepatitis	Radiation hepatitis
	Steatohepatitis

* See also changes in the current SMQ version.

Search 2.4: SMQ code 20000011 *
Sub-SMQ *Liver neoplasms malignant and unspecified*

Sub-SMQ Liver neoplasms malignant and unspecified MedDRA v8.0	Sub-SMQ Liver neoplasms malignant and unspecified MedDRA v18.0
	Sub-SMQ *Liver malignant tumours*
	Hepatic angiosarcoma
	Hepatic cancer
Hepatic cancer metastatic	Hepatic cancer metastatic
	Hepatic cancer recurrent
Hepatic cancer stage I	Hepatic cancer stage I
Hepatic cancer stage II	Hepatic cancer stage II
Hepatic cancer stage III	Hepatic cancer stage III
Hepatic cancer stage IV	Hepatic cancer stage IV
	Hepatobiliary cancer
	Hepatobiliary cancer in situ
	Hepatoblastoma
	Hepatoblastoma recurrent
Hepatobiliary carcinoma in situ	
Hepatic neoplasm	
Hepatic neoplasm malignant	
Hepatic neoplasm malignant non-resectable	
Hepatic neoplasm malignant recurrent	
Hepatic neoplasm malignant resectable	
Hepatobiliary neoplasm	
Hepatoblastoma	
	Hepatocellular carcinoma

Sub-SMQ Liver neoplasms malignant and unspecified MedDRA v8.0	Sub-SMQ Liver neoplasms malignant and unspecified MedDRA v18.0
Hepatoblastoma recurrent	
	Liver ablation
Liver carcinoma ruptured	Liver carcinoma ruptured
Malignant hepatobiliary neoplasm	
Mixed hepatocellular cholangiocarcinoma	Mixed hepatocellular cholangiocarcinoma
	Sub-SMQ *Liver tumours of unspecified malignancy*
	Hepatic neoplasm
	Hepatobiliary neoplasm

* See also changes in the current SMQ version.

Search 2.5: SMQ code 20000012 *
Sub-SMQ *Liver neoplasms benign*

Sub-SMQ Liver neoplasms benign MedDRA v8.0	Sub-SMQ Liver neoplasms, benign (incl cysts and polyps) MedDRA v18.0
Benign hepatic neoplasm	Benign hepatic neoplasm
Focal nodular hyperplasia	Focal nodular hyperplasia
Haemangioma of liver	Haemangioma of liver
	Haemorrhagic hepatic cyst
Hepatic adenoma	Hepatic adenoma
Hepatic cyst	Hepatic cyst
Hepatic cyst ruptured	Hepatic cyst ruptured
Hepatic haemangioma rupture	Hepatic haemangioma rupture

* See also changes in the current SMQ version.

Search 2.6: SMQ code 20000013 *
Sub-SMQ *Hepatic failure, fibrosis and cirrhosis and other liver damage-related conditions*

Sub-SMQ Hepatic failure, fibrosis and cirrhosis and other liver damage related conditions MedDRA v8.0	Sub-SMQ Hepatic failure, fibrosis and cirrhosis and other liver damage-related conditions MedDRA v18.0
	Acute hepatic failure
	Acute yellow liver atrophy
	Anorectal varices
	Anorectal varices haemorrhage
Ascites	Ascites
Asterixis	Asterixis

APPENDIX 2. EXAMPLES OF SMQ DEVELOPMENT

Sub-SMQ Hepatic failure, fibrosis and cirrhosis and other liver damage related conditions MedDRA v8.0	Sub-SMQ Hepatic failure, fibrosis and cirrhosis and other liver damage-related conditions MedDRA v18.0
	Bacterascites
Biliary cirrhosis	Biliary cirrhosis
Biliary cirrhosis primary	Biliary cirrhosis primary
Biliary fibrosis	Biliary fibrosis
	Cholestatic liver injury
	Chronic hepatic failure
Coma hepatic	Coma hepatic
	Cryptogenic cirrhosis
	Diabetic hepatopathy
	Drug-induced liver injury
	Duodenal varices
	Gallbladder varices
	Gastric variceal injection
	Gastric variceal ligation
	Gastric varices
	Gastric varices haemorrhage
Hepatectomy	Hepatectomy
Hepatic atrophy	Hepatic atrophy
	Hepatic calcification
Hepatic cirrhosis	Hepatic cirrhosis
Hepatic encephalopathy	Hepatic encephalopathy
	Hepatic encephalopathy prophylaxis
Hepatic failure	Hepatic failure
Hepatic fibrosis	Hepatic fibrosis
	Hepatic hydrothorax
	Hepatic infiltration eosinophilic
Hepatic lesion	Hepatic lesion
Hepatic necrosis	Hepatic necrosis
Hepatic steatosis	Hepatic steatosis
	Hepatitis fulminant
Hepatobiliary disease	Hepatobiliary disease
Hepatocellular damage	
Hepatocellular foamy cell syndrome	Hepatocellular foamy cell syndrome
	Hepatocellular injury
Hepatopulmonary syndrome	Hepatopulmonary syndrome

Sub-SMQ Hepatic failure, fibrosis and cirrhosis and other liver damage related conditions MedDRA v8.0	Sub-SMQ Hepatic failure, fibrosis and cirrhosis and other liver damage-related conditions MedDRA v18.0
Hepatorenal failure	Hepatorenal failure
Hepatorenal syndrome	Hepatorenal syndrome
Hepatotoxicity	Hepatotoxicity
	Intestinal varices
	Intrahepatic portal hepatic venous fistula
Liver and small intestine transplant	Liver and small intestine transplant
Liver disorder	Liver disorder
	Liver injury
Liver operation	Liver operation
Liver transplant	Liver transplant
Lupoid hepatic cirrhosis	Lupoid hepatic cirrhosis
	Minimal hepatic encephalopathy
	Mixed liver injury
Nodular regenerative hyperplasia	Nodular regenerative hyperplasia
Non-alcoholic steatohepatitis	Non-alcoholic steatohepatitis
Oedema due to hepatic disease	Oedema due to hepatic disease
Oesophageal varices haemorrhage	Oesophageal varices haemorrhage
	Peripancreatic varices
	Peritoneovenous shunt
	Portal fibrosis
Portal hypertension	Portal hypertension
	Portal hypertensive enteropathy
	Portal hypertensive gastropathy
	Portal shunt
Portal triaditis	
	Portal vein cavernous transformation
	Portal vein dilatation
	Portopulmonary hypertension
Renal and liver transplant	Renal and liver transplant
	Retrograde portal vein flow
Reye's syndrome	Reye's syndrome
	Reynold's syndrome
	Small-for-size liver syndrome
Spider naevus	Spider naevus
	Splenic varices

APPENDIX 2. EXAMPLES OF SMQ DEVELOPMENT

Sub-SMQ Hepatic failure, fibrosis and cirrhosis and other liver damage related conditions MedDRA v8.0	Sub-SMQ Hepatic failure, fibrosis and cirrhosis and other liver damage-related conditions MedDRA v18.0
	Splenic varices haemorrhage
	Spontaneous intrahepatic portosystemic venous shunt
	Steatohepatitis
	Stomal varices
	Subacute hepatic failure
Varices oesophageal	Varices oesophageal
	Varicose veins of abdominal wall

* See also changes in the current SMQ version.

Search 2.7: SMQ code 20000014 *
Sub-SMQ Congenital, familial, neonatal and genetic disorders of the liver

Sub-SMQ Congenital, familial, neonatal and genetic disorders of the liver MedDRA v8.0	Sub-SMQ Congenital, familial, neonatal and genetic disorders of the liver MedDRA 18.0
Accessory liver lobe	Accessory liver lobe
Alagille syndrome	Alagille syndrome
Cerebrohepatorenal syndrome	Cerebrohepatorenal syndrome
Congenital absence of bile ducts	Congenital absence of bile ducts
Congenital cystic disease of liver	Congenital cystic disease of liver
Congenital hepatic fibrosis	Congenital hepatic fibrosis
Congenital hepatobiliary anomaly	Congenital hepatobiliary anomaly
Congenital hepatomegaly	Congenital hepatomegaly
	Cystic fibrosis hepatic disease
Dilatation intrahepatic duct congenital	Dilatation intrahepatic duct congenital
	Glycogen storage disease type I
	Glycogen storage disease type III
	Glycogen storage disease type IV
	Glycogen storage disease type VI
Hepatitis neonatal	Hepatitis neonatal
Hepatocellular damage neonatal	Hepatocellular damage neonatal
Hepato-lenticular degeneration	Hepato-lenticular degeneration
Hepatosplenomegaly neonatal	Hepatosplenomegaly neonatal
Hereditary haemochromatosis	Hereditary haemochromatosis

Sub-SMQ Congenital, familial, neonatal and genetic disorders of the liver MedDRA v8.0	Sub-SMQ Congenital, familial, neonatal and genetic disorders of the liver MedDRA 18.0
Hyperbilirubinaemia neonatal	Hyperbilirubinaemia neonatal
Jaundice neonatal	Jaundice neonatal
Kernicterus	Kernicterus
Neonatal cholestasis	Neonatal cholestasis
Neonatal hepatomegaly	Neonatal hepatomegaly
Polycystic liver disease	Polycystic liver disease
Porphyria acute	Porphyria acute
Porphyria non-acute	Porphyria non-acute
	Progressive familial intrahepatic cholestasis
Pseudoporphyria	

* See also changes in the current SMQ version.

Search 2.8: SMQ code 20000015 *
Sub-SMQ *Possibly liver-related coagulation and bleeding disturbances*

Sub-SMQ Possibly liver related coagulation and bleeding disturbances MedDRA v8.0	Sub-SMQ Liver-related coagulation and bleeding disturbances MedDRA v18.0
	Acquired antithrombin III deficiency
Antithrombin III decreased	Antithrombin III decreased
Blood fibrinogen abnormal	Blood fibrinogen abnormal
Blood fibrinogen decreased	Blood fibrinogen decreased
Blood thrombin abnormal	Blood thrombin abnormal
Blood thrombin decreased	Blood thrombin decreased
Blood thromboplastin abnormal	Blood thromboplastin abnormal
Blood thromboplastin decreased	Blood thromboplastin decreased
Coagulation factor decreased	Coagulation factor decreased
Coagulation factor IX level abnormal	Coagulation factor IX level abnormal
Coagulation factor IX level decreased	Coagulation factor IX level decreased
Coagulation factor V level abnormal	Coagulation factor V level abnormal
Coagulation factor V level decreased	Coagulation factor V level decreased
Coagulation factor VII level abnormal	Coagulation factor VII level abnormal
Coagulation factor VII level decreased	Coagulation factor VII level decreased
Coagulation factor X level abnormal	Coagulation factor X level abnormal
Coagulation factor X level decreased	Coagulation factor X level decreased
	Hyperfibrinolysis
	Hypocoagulable state

Sub-SMQ Possibly liver related coagulation and bleeding disturbances MedDRA v8.0	Sub-SMQ Liver-related coagulation and bleeding disturbances MedDRA v18.0
	Hypofibrinogenaemia
	Hypoprothrombinaemia
	Hypothrombinaemia
	Hypothromboplastinaemia
International normalised ratio abnormal	International normalised ratio abnormal
International normalised ratio decreased	International normalised ratio increased
Protein C decreased	Protein C decreased
Protein S abnormal	Protein S abnormal
Protein S decreased	Protein S decreased
Prothrombin level abnormal	Prothrombin level abnormal
Prothrombin level decreased	Prothrombin level decreased
Prothrombin time abnormal	Prothrombin time abnormal
Prothrombin time prolonged	Prothrombin time prolonged
Prothrombin time ratio abnormal	Prothrombin time ratio abnormal
Prothrombin time ratio decreased	Prothrombin time ratio increased
Thrombin time abnormal	Thrombin time abnormal
Thrombin time prolonged	Thrombin time prolonged

* See also changes in the current SMQ version.

Search 2.9: SMQ code 20000016 *
Sub-SMQ *Liver infections*

Sub-SMQ Liver infections MedDRA v8.0	Sub-SMQ Liver infections MedDRA v18.0
	Acute hepatitis B
	Acute hepatitis C
Adenoviral hepatitis	Adenoviral hepatitis
Amoebic liver abscess	
Anti-HBc antibody positive	
Anti-HBe antibody positive	
Anti-HBc IgM antibody positive	
Anti-HBs antibody positive	
	Asymptomatic viral hepatitis
	Chronic hepatitis B
	Chronic hepatitis C
Congenital hepatitis B infection	Congenital hepatitis B infection
Cytomegalovirus hepatitis	Cytomegalovirus hepatitis
Gianotti-Crosti syndrome	Gianotti-Crosti syndrome

Sub-SMQ Liver infections MedDRA v8.0	Sub-SMQ Liver infections MedDRA v18.0
	HBV-DNA polymerase increased
	Hepatic amoebiasis
Hepatic candidiasis	Hepatic candidiasis
Hepatic cyst infection	Hepatic cyst infection
Hepatic echinococciasis	Hepatic echinococciasis
Hepatic infection	Hepatic infection
	Hepatic infection bacterial
	Hepatic infection fungal
	Hepatic infection helminthic
Hepatitis A	Hepatitis A
Hepatitis A antibody abnormal	Hepatitis A antibody abnormal
Hepatitis A antibody positive	Hepatitis A antibody positive
Hepatitis A antigen positive	Hepatitis A antigen positive
Hepatitis A positive	
	Hepatitis A virus test positive
Hepatitis B	Hepatitis B
Hepatitis B antibody abnormal	Hepatitis B antibody abnormal
Hepatitis B antibody positive	Hepatitis B antibody positive
	Hepatitis B core antibody positive
Hepatitis B core antigen positive	Hepatitis B core antigen positive
Hepatitis B DNA assay positive	Hepatitis B DNA assay positive
Hepatitis B positive	
	Hepatitis B DNA increased
	Hepatitis B e antibody positive
Hepatitis B e antigen positive	Hepatitis B e antigen positive
	Hepatitis B surface antibody positive
Hepatitis B surface antigen positive	Hepatitis B surface antigen positive
	Hepatitis B virus test positive
Hepatitis C	Hepatitis C
Hepatitis C antibody positive	Hepatitis C antibody positive
	Hepatitis C RNA increased
Hepatitis C positive	
Hepatitis C RNA positive	Hepatitis C RNA positive
	Hepatitis C virus test positive
Hepatitis D	Hepatitis D
Hepatitis D antibody positive	Hepatitis D antibody positive
Hepatitis D antigen positive	Hepatitis D antigen positive

APPENDIX 2. EXAMPLES OF SMQ DEVELOPMENT

Sub-SMQ Liver infections MedDRA v8.0	Sub-SMQ Liver infections MedDRA v18.0 *
Hepatitis D RNA positive	Hepatitis D RNA positive
	Hepatitis D virus test positive
Hepatitis E	Hepatitis E
Hepatitis E antibody abnormal	Hepatitis E antibody abnormal
Hepatitis E antibody positive	Hepatitis E antibody positive
Hepatitis E antigen positive	Hepatitis E antigen positive
	Hepatitis E virus test positive
Hepatitis F	Hepatitis F
Hepatitis G	Hepatitis G
Hepatitis H	Hepatitis H
Hepatitis infectious	Hepatitis infectious
Hepatitis infectious mononucleosis	Hepatitis infectious mononucleosis
Hepatitis mumps	Hepatitis mumps
Hepatitis non-A non-B	Hepatitis non-A non-B
Hepatitis non-A non-B non-C	Hepatitis non-A non-B non-C
Hepatitis post transfusion	Hepatitis post transfusion
Hepatitis syphilitic	Hepatitis syphilitic
Hepatitis toxoplasmal	Hepatitis toxoplasmal
Hepatitis viral	Hepatitis viral
	Hepatitis viral test positive
Hepatobiliary infection	Hepatobiliary infection
Hepatosplenic candidiasis	Hepatosplenic candidiasis
	Herpes simplex hepatitis
Liver abscess	Liver abscess
Perihepatitis gonococcal	
	Perinatal HBV infection
Portal pyaemia	Portal pyaemia
Schistosomiasis liver	Schistosomiasis liver
	Sustained viral response
Viral hepatitis carrier	Viral hepatitis carrier
Weil's disease	Weil's disease
	Withdrawal hepatitis

* See also changes in the current SMQ version.

Search 2.10: SMQ code 2000001 *
Sub-SMQ *Events specifically reported as alcohol-related*

Sub-SMQ Events specifically reported as alcohol related MedDRA v8.0	Sub-SMQ Hepatic disorders specifically reported as alcohol-related MedDRA v18.0
Alcoholic liver disease	Alcoholic liver disease
Cirrhosis alcoholic	Cirrhosis alcoholic
Fatty liver alcoholic	Fatty liver alcoholic
Hepatitis alcoholic	Hepatitis alcoholic
Zieve syndrome	Zieve syndrome

* See also changes in the current SMQ version.

Search 2.11: SMQ code 20000018 *
Sub-SMQ *Pregnancy-related hepatic disorders*

Sub-SMQ Pregnancy related hepatic disorders MedDRA v8.0	Sub-SMQ Pregnancy-related hepatic disorders MedDRA v18.0
Acute fatty liver of pregnancy	Acute fatty liver of pregnancy
Cholestasis of pregnancy	Cholestasis of pregnancy

* See also changes in the current SMQ version.

Search 3

Search 3.1: SMQ code 20000006
Sub-SMQ *Possibly drug related hepatic disorders – comprehensive search*

All Terms of searches 2.1 to 2.6 and 2.8.

Search 3.2: SMQ code 20000007
Sub-SMQ *Possibly drug related hepatic disorders – severe events only*

All Terms of searches 2.3 to 2.6.

References:

1. Introductory guide: Standardised MedDRA Queries (SMQ) Version 18.0, MSSO-DI-6226-18.0.0, March 2015. See the relevant version on www.meddra.org

APPENDIX 3.

COMMUNICATION OF SEARCH RESULTS

This appendix contains a template for communicating the results of a search, as described in Chapter V. The various sections of the template should be considered for completeness of a report, but numbering and content may be modified to fit the circumstances of the report. It is appropriate to provide a rationale for modifications to the content or format of the report.

Table A.3.1. Communication of search results

Sections	Content to consider
Executive summary	Summary of question
	Origin of question
	Overview of search strategy
	Overview of results
	Overview of conclusion
1. Background for question	
1.a. Introduction	Specific query
	Source of request
	Historical aspects, relevant time window for query
	Objective of report
	Relationship of query to any related conditions in the reference safety information
1.b. Medicinal product	Indication
	Formulation
	Posology
	Mechanism of action
	Stage of development/marketing status
	Product label information (investigator brochure/prescribing information)
	Population exposure (split by clinical trial exposure and post-marketing, if appropriate)
1.c. Medical condition of interest	Natural history of condition
	Symptoms, signs
	Other treatment(s)

Sections	Content to consider
	Does definition in *Introductory guide for SMQs* [1] match the condition of interest?
2. Methods	
2.a. Search and selection strategy	Scope of query
2.b. MedDRA version of SMQ	Address any differences between MedDRA version of data and version of SMQ used for query
2.c. SMQ utilized	Name of level 1/parent SMQ
	If hierarchical SMQ, name sub-SMQs
	Specify narrow or broad scope
	If algorithmic SMQ or SMQ with term weightings, whether these were applied
2.d. SMQ modified	If modified, describe changes
2.e. Data sources	ICSRs from organized data collection schemes (e.g. clinical trials, observational studies) and/or spontaneous sources.
	Countries
	Serious/non-serious
	Health-care professional/non-health-care professional reports
	Causality
	Any limitations of data
	Multiple sources: co-development/in-licensing/epidemiology. Differences in coding conventions, data migration, mapping from other coding terminologies, MedDRA versioning practices
2.f. Medical assessment	Process of medical review: any validation or triage, filters applied, processes for "noise" reduction
3. Results of query	
3.a. Overview	Summary: number of cases, time window, type of data retrieved
3.b. Cases presentation	Summary of relevant cases, cases to be excluded (with rationale). Limitations of data
3.c. Summary of data	Consolidate query findings
3.d. Additional relevant information	
4. Discussion and conclusion	
5. References	References from literature if relevant

References:

1. Introductory guide for Standardised MedDRA Queries (SMQs), Version 18.1, MSSO-DI-6226-18.1.0, September 2015. See the relevant version on www.meddra.org